T0383247

Cancer Emergencies, Part I

Guest Editors

MOHAMUD DAYA, MD, MS
CHARLES R. THOMAS, JR., MD

EMERGENCY MEDICINE CLINICS OF NORTH AMERICA

www.emed.theclinics.com

Consulting Editor
AMAL MATTU, MD

May 2009 • Volume 27 • Number 2

SAUNDERS an imprint of ELSEVIER, Inc.

W.B. SAUNDERS COMPANY

A Division of Elsevier Inc.

1600 John F. Kennedy Boulevard • Suite 1800 • Philadelphia, Pennsylvania 19103-2899

http://www.theclinics.com

EMERGENCY MEDICINE CLINICS OF NORTH AMERICA Volume 27, Number 2
May 2009 ISSN 0733-8627, ISBN-13: 978-1-4377-0470-9, ISBN-10: 1-4377-0470-0

Editor: Patrick Manley
Developmental Editor: Theresa Collier

© **2009 Elsevier ■ All rights reserved.**

This journal and the individual contributions contained in it are protected under copyright by Elsevier, and the following terms and conditions apply to their use:

Photocopying
Single photocopies of single articles may be made for personal use as allowed by national copyright laws. Permission of the Publisher and payment of a fee is required for all other photocopying, including multiple or systematic copying, copying for advertising or promotional purposes, resale, and all forms of document delivery. Special rates are available for educational institutions that wish to make photocopies for non-profit educational classroom use. For information on how to seek permission visit www.elsevier.com/permissions or call: (+44) 1865 843830 (UK)/(+1) 215 239 3804 (USA).

Derivative Works
Subscribers may reproduce tables of contents or prepare lists of articles including abstracts for internal circulation within their institutions. Permission of the Publisher is required for resale or distribution outside the institution. Permission of the Publisher is required for all other derivative works, including compilations and translations (please consult www.elsevier.com/permissions).

Electronic Storage or Usage
Permission of the Publisher is required to store or use electronically any material contained in this journal, including any article or part of an article (please consult www.elsevier.com/permissions). Except as outlined above, no part of this publication may be reproduced, stored in a retrieval system or transmitted in any form or by any means, electronic, mechanical, photocopying, recording or otherwise, without prior written permission of the Publisher.

Notice
No responsibility is assumed by the Publisher for any injury and/or damage to persons or property as a matter of products liability, negligence or otherwise, or from any use or operation of any methods, products, instructions or ideas contained in the material herein. Because of rapid advances in the medical sciences, in particular, independent verification of diagnoses and drug dosages should be made.

Although all advertising material is expected to conform to ethical (medical) standards, inclusion in this publication does not constitute a guarantee or endorsement of the quality or value of such product or of the claims made of it by its manufacturer.

Emergency Medicine Clinics of North America (ISSN 0733-8627) is published quarterly by Elsevier Inc., 360 Park Avenue South, New York, NY, 10010-1710. Months of issue are February, May, August, and November. Business and Editorial Offices: 1600 John F. Kennedy Boulevard, Suite 1800, Philadelphia, PA 19103-2899. Customer Service Office: 6277 Sea Harbor Drive, Orlando, FL 32887-4800. Periodicals postage paid at New York, NY, and additional mailing offices. Subscription prices are $118.00 per year (US students), $229.00 per year (US individuals), $373.00 per year (US institutions), $167.00 per year (international students), $328.00 per year (international individuals), $450.00 per year (international institutions), $167.00 per year (Canadian students), $282.00 per year (Canadian individuals), and $450.00 per year (Canadian institutions). International air speed delivery is included in all *Clinics'* subscription prices. All prices are subject to change without notice. **POSTMASTER:** Send address changes to *Emergency Medicine Clinics of North America*, Elsevier Periodicals Customer Service, 11830 Westline Industrial Drive, St. Louis, MO 63146. Customer Service (orders, claims, online, change of address): Elsevier Periodicals Customer Service, 11830 Westline Industrial Drive, St. Louis, MO 63146. Tel: 1-800-654-2452 (U.S. and Canada); 314-453-7041 (outside U.S. and Canada). Fax: 314-453-5170. E-mail: journalscustomerservice-usa@elsevier.com (for print support); journalsonline support-usa@elsevier.com (for online support).

Reprints. For copies of 100 or more of articles in this publication, please contact the Commercial Reprints Department, Elsevier Inc., 360 Park Avenue South, New York, NY 10010-1710. Tel.: 212-633-3812; Fax: 212-462-1935; E-mail: reprints@elsevier.com.

Emergency Medicine Clinics of North America is covered in *MEDLINE/PubMed (Index Medicus), Current Contents/Clinical Medicine, EMBASE/Excerpta Medica, BIOSIS, SciSearch, CINAHL, ISI/BIOMED,* and *Research Alert.*

Printed and bound by CPI Group (UK) Ltd, Croydon, CR0 4YY
Transferred to Digital Print 2011

Contributors

CONSULTING EDITOR

AMAL MATTU, MD, FAAEM, FACEP
Associate Professor and Program Director, Department of Emergency Medicine,
University of Maryland School of Medicine, Baltimore, Maryland

GUEST EDITORS

MOHAMUD DAYA, MD, MS
Associate Professor and Vice Chair, Department of Emergency Medicine, Oregon Health
& Science University, Portland, Oregon

CHARLES R. THOMAS, Jr., MD
Professor and Chair, Department of Radiation Medicine, Oregon Health & Science
University, Portland, Oregon

AUTHORS

DAVID E. ADELBERG, MD
Senior Fellow, Medical Oncology Branch, National Cancer Institute, Bethesda, Maryland

ANDREA BEZJAK, MD, MSc, FRCPC
Associate Professor, Department of Radiation Oncology, University of Toronto, Princess
Margaret Hospital, Toronto, Ontario, Canada

MICHAEL R. BISHOP, MD
Experimental Transplantation and Immunology Branch, National Cancer Institute,
Bethesda, Maryland

JEFFREY A. BOGART, MD
Professor and Chairman, Department of Radiation Oncology, State University of New York
Upstate Medical University, Syracuse, New York

PLACID BONE, MD
Interfaith Medical Center, Brooklyn, New York

RAHUL R. CHOPRA, MD
Department of Radiation Oncology, State University of New York Upstate Medical
University, Syracuse, New York

DENISE M. DAMEK, MD
Associate Professor, Neurology and Neurosurgery, University of Colorado Denver School
of Medicine, Neuro-Oncology Program, Aurora, Colorado

PAUL L. DeSANDRE, DO
Assistant Professor, Emergency Medicine, Albert Einstein College of Medicine; Attending Physician, Emergency Medicine, Hospice and Palliative Medicine, Beth Israel Medical Center, New York, New York

MELISSA L. GIVENS, MD, MPH
Emergency Medicine Residency Director, Department of Emergency Medicine, Carl R. Darnall Army Medical Center, Fort Hood, Texas; Assistant Professor, Department of Military and Emergency Medicine, Uniformed Services University of the Health Sciences, Bethesda, Maryland

ROBERT F. KACPROWICZ, MD
Program Director, San Antonio Uniformed Services Health Education Consortium Residency in Emergency Medicine, San Antonio, Texas; Assistant Clinical Professor, Department of Emergency Medicine, University of New Mexico School of Medicine, Albuquerque, New Mexico; Department of Emergency Medicine, Wilford Hall USAF Medical Center, Lackland AFB, Texas

JEREMY D. LLOYD, MD
Co-Director of Medical Student and Intern Education, San Antonio Uniformed Services Health Education Consortium Residency in Emergency Medicine, San Antonio; Department of Emergency Medicine, Wilford Hall USAF Medical Center, Lackland AFB, Texas

ANDREW N. NEMECEK, MD
Assistant Professor, Department of Neurological Surgery, Oregon Health and Science University, Portland, Oregon

TAMMIE E. QUEST, MD
Associate Professor, Department of Emergency Medicine, Emory University School of Medicine, Atlanta, Georgia

DAWN FELCH RONDEAU, MS, ACNP, FNP
Senior Instructor, Department of Emergency Medicine, Oregon Health and Science University, Portland, Oregon; Adjunct Faculty, Department of Nursing, Washington State University, Vancouver, Washington

TERRI A. SCHMIDT, MD, MS
Professor, Department of Emergency Medicine, Oregon Health and Science University, Portland, Oregon

HAI SUN, MD, PhD
Resident, Department of Neurological Surgery, Oregon Health and Science University, Portland, Oregon

YAEL R. TAUB, MD
Attending Physician, Department of Emergency Medicine, University Hospitals Case Medical Center; Assistant Professor, Department of Emergency Medicine, Case Western Reserve University School of Medicine, Cleveland, Ohio

PIERRE R. THEODORE, MD
Van Auken Endowed Chair; Assistant Professor, Division of Thoracic Surgery, Department of Surgery, University of California at San Francisco, San Francisco, California

JONATHAN F. WAN, BASc, MD, FRCPC
Fellow, Department of Radiation Oncology, University of Toronto, Princess Margaret Hospital, Toronto, Ontario; Assistant Professor, Department of Radiation Oncology, McGill University, Montreal General Hospital, Montreal, Quebec, Canada

JOY WETHERN, DO, FACEP, FACMT
Senior Resident, Department of Emergency Medicine, Carl R. Darnall Army Medical Center, Fort Hood, Texas

ROBERT W. WOLFORD, MD, MMM
Director of Clinical Operations, Department of Emergency Medicine, University Hospitals Case Medical Center; Associate Professor, Department of Emergency Medicine, Case Western Reserve University School of Medicine, Cleveland, Ohio

Contributors

Contents

> Patients and families struggling with cancer fear pain more than any other physical symptom. There are also significant barriers to optimal pain management in the emergency setting, including lack of knowledge, inexperienced clinicians, myths about addiction, and fears of complications after discharge. In this article, we review the assessment and management options for cancer-related pain based on the World Health Organization (WHO) 3-step approach.

> Malignant epidural spinal cord compression (MESCC) is a common neurologic complication of cancer. MESCC is a medical emergency that needs rapid diagnosis and treatment to prevent paraplegia. Patients with malignancy who present with new onset of neurologic signs and symptoms should undergo emergent evaluation including magnetic resonance imaging of the entire spine. If MESCC is diagnosed, corticosteroids should be administered. Simultaneously, spine surgery and oncology teams should be immediately consulted. If indicated, patients should undergo maximal tumor resection and stabilization, followed by postoperative radiotherapy. Emerging treatment options such as stereotactic radiosurgery and vertebroplasty may be able to provide some symptomatic relief for patients who are not surgical candidates.

> Neurologic symptoms commonly occur in oncology patients, and in some cases they may be the presenting symptom of malignancy. Cancer-related neurologic syndromes are rarely pathognomonic and must be differentiated from other benign or serious conditions. This article reviews common neuro-oncologic syndromes that may lead to urgent evaluation in the emergency department, including cerebral edema, altered mental status, seizures, acute stroke, leptomeningeal metastases, and paraneoplastic neurologic syndromes.

Acute obstruction of the airway in the emergent situation results from a wide variety of malignant and benign disease processes. Acute management involves establishing a secure and patent route for adequate gas exchange. This requires rapid determination of the location of the obstruction and nature of the obstruction followed by a thoughtful management approach based on findings. Difficult anatomy, hemorrhage, dense secretions, inflammation, and bulky tumor mass can significantly complicate the task of clearing the airway. Obstruction of the central airways by malignant tumor is associated with poor prognosis, but quality of life is considerably improved by restoration of adequate central airways. For both the patient and the clinician, the presentation can be frightening, and advanced interventional pulmonary/endobronchial techniques are required to achieve prompt relief of symptoms. The alleviation of central airway obstruction by tumor is most often palliative, with improvement of quality of life the primary goal rather than cure. This review will cover covers an approach to the patient with airway obstruction that results from malignancy involving the trachea or proximal bronchial tree and affecting gas exchange.

Superior vena cava syndrome (SVCS) is a common complication of malignancy. The epidemiology, presentation, and diagnostic evaluation of patients presenting with the syndrome are reviewed. Management options including chemotherapy and radiation therapy (RT) and the role of endovascular stents are discussed along with the evidence for each of the therapeutic options.

A thorough working knowledge of the diagnosis and treatment of life-threatening electrolyte abnormalities in cancer patients, especially hyponatremia, hypoglycemia, and hypercalcemia, is essential to the successful practice of emergency medicine. Although most minor abnormalities have no specific treatment, severe clinical manifestations of several notable electrolytes occur with significant frequency in the setting of malignancy. The treatment of life-threatening electrolyte abnormalities is reviewed here. Promising future treatments directed at the underlying physiology are also introduced.

Normal function of the adrenal gland can be disrupted not only by metastases of nonadrenal cancers but also by their treatment. In addition, tumors of the adrenal gland itself can cause disease by hypersecretion of a variety of hormones, adrenal gland destruction with inadequate production of cortisol, and by metastasis to other sites. Although rare, abnormal adrenal function should be considered in the appropriate clinical settings as failure to recognize and treat can result in significant morbidity and mortality. The adrenal "incidentaloma" is a frequent finding of abdominal radiologic studies. All patients with an unexpected adrenal mass should be referred for further evaluation.

Acute renal failure (ARF) can be one of the many complications associated with malignancy and, unfortunately, often harbors a worse prognosis for the afflicted patient. Insult to the kidneys can occur for a variety of reasons in the oncologic patient. This article focuses on several of these etiologies, such as tumor lysis syndrome (TLS) and thrombotic microangiopathy (TMA), which are unique threats faced by the oncologic patient.

TREATMENT-RELATED COMPLICATIONS PRESENTING TO THE EMERGENCY DEPARTMENT

In the modern age of cancer therapy, advances in the multidisciplinary management of cancer have resulted in increased rates of survivorship. Radiation therapy (RT) toxicity must be tempered with the desire to achieve dose escalation to provide the best chance of long-term cure. This article is designed to acquaint emergency medicine physicians with common, expected, and potential acute and late complications of RT.

As a vast majority of oncologic treatments are being administered in the outpatient setting, emergency department (ED) physicians are increasingly encountering patients who present with a wide array of toxicities that are a direct effect of chemotherapy. This review aims to highlight the most often encountered and clinically relevant toxicities of the more commonly administered chemotherapeutic drugs. In addition, because stem cell transplantation is being used increasingly for various malignancies, a brief introduction to post-transplant complications is included.

THE CLINICS ARE NOW AVAILABLE ONLINE!

Access your subscription at:
www.theclinics.com

GOAL STATEMENT
The goal of *Emergency Medicine Clinics of North America* is to keep practicing physicians up to date with current clinical practice in emergency medicine by providing timely articles reviewing the state of the art in patient care.

ACCREDITATION
The *Emergency Medical Clinics of North America* is planned and implemented in accordance with the Essential Areas and Policies of the Accreditation Council for Continuing Medical Education (ACCME) through the joint sponsorship of the University of Virginia School of Medicine and Elsevier. The University of Virginia School of Medicine is accredited by the ACCME to provide continuing medical education for physicians.

The University of Virginia School of Medicine designates this educational activity for a maximum of 15 *AMA PRA Category 1 Credits*™ for each issue, 60 credits per year. Physicians should only claim credit commensurate with the extent of their participation in the activity.

The American Medical Association has determined that physicians not licensed in the US who participate in this CME activity are eligible for a maximum of 15 *AMA PRA Category 1 Credits*™ for each issue, 60 credits per year.

The *Emergency Medicine Clinics of North America* CME program is approved by the American College of Emergency Physicians for 60 hours of ACEP Category I credit per year.

Credit can be earned by reading the text material, taking the CME examination online at http://www.theclinics.com/home/cme, and completing the evaluation. After taking the test, you will be required to review any and all incorrect answers. Following completion of the test and evaluation, your credit will be awarded and you may print your certificate.

FACULTY DISCLOSURE/CONFLICT OF INTEREST
The University of Virginia School of Medicine, as an ACCME accredited provider, endorses and strives to comply with the Accreditation Council for Continuing Medical Education (ACCME) Standards of Commercial Support, Commonwealth of Virginia statutes, University of Virginia policies and procedures, and associated federal and private regulations and guidelines on the need for disclosure and monitoring of proprietary and financial interests that may affect the scientific integrity and balance of content delivered in continuing medical education activities under our auspices.

The University of Virginia School of Medicine requires that all CME activities accredited through this institution be developed independently and be scientifically rigorous, balanced and objective in the presentation/discussion of its content, theories and practices.

All authors/editors participating in an accredited CME activity are expected to disclose to the readers relevant financial relationships with commercial entities occurring within the past 12 months (such as grants or research support, employee, consultant, stock holder, member of speakers bureau, etc.). The University of Virginia School of Medicine will employ appropriate mechanisms to resolve potential conflicts of interest to maintain the standards of fair and balanced education to the reader. Questions about specific strategies can be directed to the Office of Continuing Medical Education, University of Virginia School of Medicine, Charlottesville, Virginia.

The faculty and staff of the University of Virginia Office of Continuing Medical Education have no financial affiliations to disclose.

The authors/editors listed below have identified no professional or financial affiliations for themselves or their spouse/partner:
David E. Adelberg, MD; Andrea Bezjak, MD, MSc, FRCPC; Michael R. Bishop, MD; Jeffrey A. Bogart, MD; Placid A. Bone, MD; Rahul R. Chopra, MD; Denise M. Damek, MD; Paul Louis DeSandre, DO; Melissa L. Givens, MD, MPH; Robert F. Kacprowicz, MD; Jeremy D. Lloyd, MD; Patrick Manley (Acquisitions Editor); Amal Mattu, MD, FAAEM, FACEP (Consulting Editor); Andrew N. Nemecek, MD; Tammie E. Quest, MD; Dawn Felch Rondeau, MS, ACNP, FNP; Terri A. Schmidt, MD, MS; Hai Sun, MD, PhD; Yael Rena Taub, MD; Charles R. Thomas, Jr., MD (Guest Editor); Jonathan F. Wan, BASc, MD, FRCPC; Joy Wethern, DO, FACEP, FACMT; Robert W. Wolford, MD, MMM; and Bill Woods, MD (Test Author).

The authors/editors listed below have identified the following professional or financial affiliations for themselves of their spouse/partner:
Mohamud Daya, MD, MS (Guest Editor) is a consultant for Philips Medical Systems.
Pierre R. Theodore, MD serves on the Speakers Bureau for UCSF.

Disclosure of Discussion of Non-FDA Approved Uses for Pharmaceutical Products and/or Medical Devices
The University of Virginia School of Medicine, as an ACCME provider, requires that all faculty presenters identify and disclose any off-label uses for pharmaceutical and medical device products. The University of Virginia School of Medicine recommends that each physician fully review all the available data on new products or procedures prior to clinical use.

TO ENROLL
To enroll in the *Emergency Medicine Clinics of North America* Continuing Medical Education program, call customer service at 1-800-654-2452 or visit us online at www.theclinics.com/home/cme. The CME program is available to subscribers for an additional fee of $195.00.

Foreword

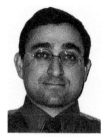

Amal Mattu, MD, FAAEM, FACEP
Consulting Editor

Anybody who has worked in emergency medicine for more than a few years has undoubtedly noticed a marked increase in the number of patients reporting a past medical history notable for cancer. This change can largely be attributable to three major factors. First, diagnostic testing for cancer has improved dramatically over the past decade, resulting in earlier detection of many neoplasms. Second, advances in therapy have increased the lifespan of many patients with cancer, turning the condition from a rapid killer in many cases into a chronic and often manageable disease. Third, advances in diagnosis and management of the two other major causes of mortality in the developed world, heart disease and stroke, are essentially allowing greater numbers of patients to live long enough to inevitably develop cancer.

The natural consequence of this is a significant increase in the number of patients presenting to our emergency departments (EDs) with either cancer-related emergencies or with other conditions in which cancer represents an important comorbidity that must be accounted for in diagnosing and treating the primary condition. It is therefore imperative that all emergency physicians gain greater familiarity with oncologic conditions and their treatments. This imperative has, in fact, encouraged an increasing number of emergency physicians to develop an academic niche focusing on oncologic emergencies. Continuing medical education conferences and publications routinely include topics related to management of solid organ and hematologic malignancies. An increasing number of research publications in emergency medicine are focusing on the diagnosis and management of oncologic emergencies. Pharmacists and toxicologists also are spending increasing amounts of time teaching about the must-know drug interactions that occur in patients taking chemotherapeutic agents. And specialists in infectious diseases are busy teaching how cancer and chemotherapy influence the evaluation and treatment of otherwise "routine" infections.

Fortunately for the readers of *Emergency Medicine Clinics of North America*, guest editors Drs. Mohamud Daya, C.R. Thomas, and David Spiro have assembled an outstanding group of authors that address all of these issues in a 2-part series. In this month's issue, they address neurologic emergencies, endocrine emergencies, metabolic and electrolyte complications, cardiovascular emergencies, airway

Emerg Med Clin N Am 27 (2009) xv–xvi
doi:10.1016/j.emc.2009.04.012
0733-8627/09/$ – see front matter © 2009 Elsevier Inc. All rights reserved.

emed.theclinics.com

complications, and toxicologic emergencies. They also address the very important issues of pain management and end-of-life care. In the August 2009 issue, they address gastrointestinal and hematologic emergencies, and they also provide several articles focused on issues relevant to pediatric patients.

Overall, the May and August 2009 issues of *Emergency Medicine Clinics* represent a comprehensive curriculum that covers the full spectrum of emergencies that ED health care providers are likely to encounter in clinical practice. These two issues represent an important contribution to education, and they are certain to improve the care of this ever-growing patient population in the ED. Our thanks go to the guest editors and their dedicated authors for this excellent work.

Amal Mattu, MD, FAAEM, FACEP
Department of Emergency Medicine
University of Maryland School of Medicine
110 S. Paca Street 6th Floor, Suite 200
Baltimore, MD 21201, USA

E-mail address:
amattu@smail.umaryland.edu (A. Mattu)

Preface

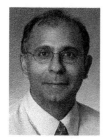 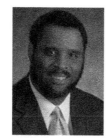

Mohamud Daya, MD, MS   Charles R. Thomas, Jr., MD
Guest Editors

Cancer will affect one in three people at some point in their lifetime and is primarily a disease of those over the age of 50. As emergency department (ED) physicians and providers see increasing numbers of cancer patients as the population ages, they need to be well prepared to deal with cancer-specific emergencies. Since the last clinics issue dedicated to this topic in 1993, there have been many advances in cancer treatment (palliative and curative), including more targeted therapies that will hopefully maximize benefit and reduce side effects.

This issue, the first of two, of *Emergency Medicine Clinics of North America* is dedicated to cancer emergencies and includes articles on specific presentation syndromes, such as malignant epidural spinal cord compression, superior vena cava syndrome, and airway obstruction. These reviews update the reader on evidence-based therapies for these entities and highlight the emerging role of stent therapies. This issue also includes articles dealing with the neurological, renal, and metabolic (electrolyte and adrenal) emergencies encountered in the cancer patient. Of particular interest are novel pharmacological therapies developed for the treatment of tumor lysis syndrome and the syndrome of inappropriate anti-diuretic hormone secretion. There also are dedicated articles that review the toxicities associated with cancer treatment, such as systemic anti-neoplastic and radiation therapy. Many cancer patients will present to the ED for care, and a better understanding of acute and chronic complications associated with treatment is essential. The important topic of pain management is reviewed comprehensively, using the World Health Organization template as a basis. Finally, this issue has two articles that deal with end-of-life and patient–provider communication issues in the ED. The important and complex interplay between cultural, spiritual, ethical, and interpersonal relationships are highlighted in these sections.

It has been a distinct pleasure to co-edit this issue, and we thank all the authors for their outstanding contributions. We also thank the leadership team associated with

Emerg Med Clin N Am 27 (2009) xvii–xviii
doi:10.1016/j.emc.2009.02.002
0733-8627/09/$ – see front matter © 2009 Elsevier Inc. All rights reserved.

Emergency Medicine Clinics of North America, especially Ms. Jeannette Forcina and Mr. Patrick Manley, for their guidance and assistance with this issue.

Mohamud Daya, MD, MS
Department of Emergency Medicine
Oregon Health & Science University
3181 SW Sam Jackson Park Road
Mail Code CDW-EM
Portland, OR 97239-3098

Charles R. Thomas, Jr., MD
Department of Radiation Medicine
Oregon Health & Science University
Mail Code KVP4
3181 SW Sam Jackson Park Road
Portland, OR 97239-3098

E-mail addresses:
dayam@ohsu.edu (M. Daya)
thomasch@ohsu.edu (C.R. Thomas)

Management of Cancer-Related Pain

Paul L. DeSandre, DO[a], Tammie E. Quest, MD[b,*]

KEYWORDS

- Pain • Malignant • Cancer • Opioids
- Emergency department

Patients and families struggling with cancer fear pain more than any other physical symptom. With the treatment of malignant pain remaining a challenge in the practice of oncology, the emergency department (ED) is often a place of refuge.[1] There are significant barriers to optimal pain management in the emergency setting, including lack of knowledge, inexperienced clinicians, myths about addiction, and fears of complications after discharge. These factors contribute to unnecessary suffering not only for the patient but also for family and caregivers. Malignant pain is highly responsive to medication. Adequate malignant pain control is possible in more than 90% of patients if established therapeutic approaches are applied systematically in any practice setting, including the ED.[2–7] It has been suggested that management of an acute pain crisis in a patient with advanced cancer "is as much a crisis as a code," and emergency clinicians should, and can, become comfortable caring for patients with cancer in acute pain.[8]

Patients with cancer often present to the ED because their pain is unmanageable. Although there are multiple physiologic possibilities for inadequate pain control, the emergency clinician should also be aware of the many psychosocial factors contributing to oligoanalgesia in the cancer patient. Depression, unresolved spiritual or social concerns, and misconceptions of prescribed medications may interfere with adequate treatment. With a properly focused evaluation, the treatment of unresolved pain in the cancer patient can be performed rapidly and effectively in the ED.

ASSESSMENT OF MALIGNANT PAIN

General principles of good pain assessment are particularly important in the patient presenting to the ED with malignancy. A rapid assessment of severity, character, likely etiology, timing and location, exacerbating and relieving factors, and associated symptoms provides essential information for proper management. In addition, the

[a] Department of Emergency Medicine, Beth Israel Medical Center, First Avenue, 16th Street, New York, NY 10003, USA
[b] Department of Emergency Medicine, Emory University School of Medicine, 69 Jesse Hill Jr. Drive, Atlanta, GA 30303, USA
* Corresponding author.
E-mail address: tquest@emory.edu (T.E. Quest).

Emerg Med Clin N Am 27 (2009) 179–194
doi:10.1016/j.emc.2009.01.002
0733-8627/09/$ – see front matter. Published by Elsevier Inc.

details of the history may reveal particular cancer pain syndromes, some of which require urgent diagnosis and intervention to prevent permanent functional impairment. With an adequate assessment, effective therapy can be quickly implemented in the ED.

The assessment of pain severity in cancer is the same as that of nonmalignant pain. There are several validated measures of a patient's pain experience. Although any scale is useful for a given patient as long as it is applied consistently, the preferred scale for most patients is the numerical rating scale (NRS).[9] Most commonly, this is an 11-point scale from 0 = "no pain" to 10 = "worst possible pain." For small children or patients with limited literacy, a picture scale is more successful, with the Faces Pain Scale being a well-accepted choice.[10] In the cognitively impaired patient, the 5-time observational Pain Assessment in Advanced Dementia Scale may be used.[11,12] All of these scales have been validated and have utility in the ED for the assessment of pain. It should be emphasized that pain scales are intended to provide objectivity to the experience of the patient's pain. Skepticism has no place in the assessment of suffering and may directly impair proper diagnosis and treatment. Pain can be complex, and these scales provide an objective method of evaluation to gauge treatment success. This is particularly true in acute pain.

The character and etiology of pain are described physiologically as either nociceptive or neuropathic. Cancer pain can be either or both. Nociceptive pain is a response to damaged tissue and can further be classified as either somatic (musculoskeletal/cutaneous) or visceral. Somatic pain is often described as sharp or aching and localized to the area of tissue damage. Pain secondary to bone metastasis is a classic example of somatic pain. Visceral pain is more poorly localized and can be intermittent, sometimes described as dull or cramping. Abdominal pain associated with ovarian or pancreatic cancers is characteristic. Neuropathic pain is primarily caused by nerve injury. The injury may be mechanical (eg, amputation), metabolic (eg, diabetes), inflammatory (eg, radiation), or toxic (eg, chemotherapy). Neuropathic pain is typically persistent and sometimes paroxysmal and shock-like. Normal stimulus may elicit abnormal pain responses (allodynia). A light touch, for example, may elicit searing pain. There can also be autonomic instability in the affected area, including edema or localized sweating such as that which occurs with complex reflex sympathetic dystrophy. An important treatment distinction between these types of pain is that patients with nociceptive pain are generally more responsive to opioids than are patients with neuropathic pain. Neuropathic pain often requires adjunctive nonopioid therapies for successful treatment.

Pain may rapidly change either in quality or location or may be chronic and slowly progressive. Although the alleviation of the pain crisis should always be the first priority, a search for the cause of the underlying pain ensures the most definitive treatment. Specific types of acute pain may require particular therapies for effective treatment, such as radiation therapy for bone metastasis. Likewise, a new location of pain may be the first sign of a dangerous progression of disease requiring diagnostic evaluation, such as new back pain preceding functional deficit in malignant epidural spinal cord compression. In addition to tumor progression, the aggressive treatments for malignancy may also be a cause for the patient's pain presentation. Surgical tumor resection may have predictable and self-limited associated pain, whereas chemotherapy-induced neuropathy may be less predictable and more persistent. The approach to treatment of these distinct types of pain will be quite different.

The assessment and management of chronic cancer pain (generally regarded as >3 months) can be challenging. Although similar to acute cancer pain in that either disease progression or treatment is typically responsible for the pain, these patients often carry a heavier global burden of suffering. The approach to treatment is more complex and must consider existing medications as well as other factors that may influence the approach to treatment.

Prior to diagnostic and therapeutic efforts in the ED, treatment must be guided by a clear understanding of the patient's goals of care. Some patients may not wish detailed investigations but may simply require pain treatment. Both acute and chronic cancer pain may be caused by disease progression (62%–78%), treatment (19%–25%), or unrelated (3%–10%) causes.[13] Patients who develop new pain are, therefore, reasonably anxious about disease progression. Communication should be sensitive to these concerns. The highly functional patient might have a goal of aggressively preserving function and longevity through early and aggressive diagnosis and management, whereas comfort alone may be the goal in an imminently dying patient.

The inescapable physical symptoms and the relentless awareness of the progression of the cancer contribute to physical, spiritual, social, and psychological strife. These factors all have the capacity to exacerbate the underlying pain. In addition, patients with pre-existing nonmalignant pain may come to the diagnosis of cancer already experiencing a sense of overwhelming suffering.[14] Cancer patients with pain are twice as likely to develop a psychiatric disorder, and as the disease progresses, the risk increases. The causes are multifactorial, and like pain, may be related to disease progression or treatment. Many of these disorders are amenable to treatment, which should be implemented as early as possible through proper referral and follow-up.[15] An interdisciplinary palliative care team, potentially hospice, should be involved as early as possible. Early palliative care intervention improves patient outcomes[16] and should be initiated by the emergency clinician when the need is identified. Depending on the institution and the urgency of the situation, palliative care consultation may occur in the ED, during hospitalization, or in the outpatient setting.

TREATMENT STRATEGIES
The WHO Stepladder

With a clear assessment of the details of the patient's pain, effective treatment can be rapidly implemented in the ED. In 1986 the WHO developed a 3-step ladder to guide the management of cancer pain. It was originally developed to address nociceptive pain (both somatic and visceral) but has proved useful to some degree for neuropathic pain as well. This simple and well-tested approach provides the clinician with a rational guide for the use of selected analgesics. Today, there is general consensus favoring the use of this model for all pain associated with serious illness. Management is based on the initial assessment of pain and should start at the step that corresponds to the patient's reported severity based on an NRS (0–10). Mild pain is defined as NRS 1 to 3 (step 1), moderate pain as NRS 4 to 6 (step 2), and severe pain as NRS 7 to 10 (step 3).

Step 1 analgesics
All of the nonopioid analgesics that characterize step 1 of the WHO ladder have a ceiling effect to their analgesia (a maximum dose that, if exceeded, yields no further analgesia). Acetaminophen is an effective step 1 analgesic and may be a useful coanalgesic in many situations, including headache. Its site and mechanism of action are not entirely known. It does not have significant anti-inflammatory effects and is presumed to have a central cyclo-oxygenase (COX) related mechanism. Chronic doses more than 4.0 g/24 h or acute doses more than 6.0 g/24 h are not recommended because they may cause hepatotoxicity. Hepatic disease or heavy alcohol use increases the risk further, and the maximum daily dosage may be reduced to 3.0 g/24 h.

Nonsteroidal anti-inflammatory drugs (NSAIDs, including aspirin) are also effective step 1 analgesics and may be useful coanalgesics. They work, at least in part, by inhibiting COX, the enzyme that converts arachidonic acid to prostaglandins. There are several classes of NSAIDs. Some patients respond better to one class of NSAIDs than to another, and serial "n of 1" trials may be needed to find one that is efficacious for a given patient. NSAIDs with longer half-lives are likely to enhance compliance. NSAIDs can have significant adverse effects. Gastropathy, renal failure, and inhibition of platelet aggregation can occur with any of the nonselective medications, irrespective of the route of administration. The likelihood of these adverse effects will vary among NSAID classes and may be due, in part, to their relative COX-2 selectivity. It is important to ensure adequate hydration and good urine output in patients on NSAIDs to minimize the risk of renal vasoconstrictive injury, including papillary necrosis. Nonselective medications are relatively contraindicated in the setting of significant pre-existing renal insufficiency. NSAIDs may be contraindicated if bleeding is a problem or coagulation or platelet function is impaired. Gastric cytoprotection with misoprostol or omeprazole may be needed in patients with significant risk of gastrointestinal (GI) problems. Significant risk factors include a history of gastric ulcers or bleeding, current nausea/vomiting, protein wasting, cachexia, and advanced age.

There are parenteral forms of NSAIDs now available for use. A new transdermal form of diclofenac is now available in the United States. Its efficacy has been demonstrated in osteoarthritis[17] but has not yet been studied in localized somatic cancer pain. Ketorolac is available in intravenous (IV) or intramuscular formulations. Short-term (<5 days is considered safe in healthy patients) parenteral use of this potent agent provides excellent analgesia, particularly with visceral pain, and avoids the common central nervous system (CNS) side effects of the opioid analgesics. These advantages must be carefully weighed against the GI, renal, cardiovascular, and bleeding risks for each patient before use.

Step 2 and step 3 analgesics

Step 2 and 3 analgesics involve opioid use. The clinician must have an excellent command of opioid pharmacology when using these analgesics. Step 2 agents all have aspirin or acetaminophen present in amounts that limit their dosages to 10 to 12 tablets a day. These agents have a role in moderate pain (4–7/10), but each also has side effects. Codeine derivatives tend to be constipating, and nausea is not infrequent. There are patients who lack the necessary enzyme to convert codeine to its active (morphine) moiety. Therefore, be aware of the need to change to morphine or a step 3 agent if no analgesia is seen. Effective treatment in the ED requires a clear understanding of the pharmacology, clinical setting, and adverse effects of the analgesics prescribed and knowledge of how these may vary from patient to patient.

PRINCIPLES OF OPIOID THERAPY
Opioid Pharmacology

Opioid analgesic effect correlates with maximal plasma concentration (Cmax) (**Table 1**). Once Cmax is reached, both the maximum analgesic effect and the maximum side-effect profile have been attained. All pure opioids (except methadone) follow first-order kinetics and act in a very similar pharmacologic manner. They reach their time to peak plasma concentration (Tmax) approximately 60 to 90 minutes after oral (including enteral feeding tube) administration, 30 minutes after subcutaneous or intramuscular injection or rectal administration, and 6 to 10 minutes after intravenous injection. They are eliminated from the body in a linear and predictable way, proportional to the dose. They are first conjugated in the liver, and then the kidneys excrete

Table 1	
Time to maximal concentration (Tmax)	
Route	**Time to Maximal Concentration**
Intravenous	6–10 min
Rectal/subcutaneous	30 min
Oral	60–90 min

90% to 95% of the metabolites. Their metabolic pathways do not become saturated. Because of its complicated cytochrome metabolism, methadone does not follow the first-order kinetics and should not be initiated or titrated in the ED without the consultation of the patient's primary care physician or a specialist in pain or palliative medicine. Each opioid metabolite has a half-life ($t_{1/2}$) that depends on its rate of renal clearance. When renal function is normal, codeine, hydrocodone, hydromorphone, morphine, oxycodone, and their metabolites all have effective half-lives of approximately 3 to 4 hours. When dosed repeatedly, their plasma concentrations approach a steady state after 4 to 5 half-lives. Thus, steady-state plasma concentrations are usually attained within a day.

Opioids and their metabolites are primarily excreted renally (90%–95%). Care should be taken when dosing these agents in patients with renal impairment. The clinician should take care in selecting appropriate agents in patients with renal impairment and be prepared to reduce the dose (**Tables 2** and **3**). Morphine has 2 principal metabolites: morphine-3-glucuronide and morphine-6-glucuronide. Morphine-6-glucuronide is active and has a longer half-life than that of the parent drug morphine. Consequently, when dehydration or acute or chronic renal failure impairs renal clearance, the dosing interval for morphine must be increased or the dosage size decreased to avoid excessive accumulation of active drug and metabolites.[18–20] If urine output is minimal (oliguria) or none (anuria), routine dosing should be stopped, and morphine should be administered only as needed. This is particularly important when patients are dying. Renal excretion is somewhat less of a concern with hydromorphone, but fentanyl and methadone are considered the safest choices in renal failure. Opioid metabolism is not as sensitive to hepatic compromise. However, if hepatic function becomes severely impaired, the dosing interval should be increased or the dose decreased.

Table 2			
Opioid selection in renal failure			
		Dialyzable	
Opioid	**Renal Failure**	**Parent Drug**	**Metabolites**
Methadone	Appears safe	+	+
Fentanyl	Appears safe	+/−	none
Morphine	Use with caution/dose adjust	+	+
Hydromorphone		+	+/−
Hydrocodone		+	+/−
Oxycodone		Inadequate data	Inadequate data
Codeine	Do not use	Inadequate data	Inadequate data
Meperidine		Inadequate data	Inadequate data
Propoxyphene		−	−

Table 3	
Opioid dose reduction in renal failure	
Creatinine Clearance	**Dose Reduction of Normal Dose**
>50 mL/min; normal dosing	Normal
10–50 mL/min	75% dosing
<10 mL/min	50% dosing

Opioid-Naïve Patients

Patients with severe pain who have never been on opioids will need a trial of short-acting opioids to establish their opioid needs and any possible respiratory depressive effect. Oral agonist opioids are appropriate for severe pain if time and circumstance allow. On an outpatient basis, severe pain may be treated with WHO step 3 analgesics as a reasonable first choice. If an immediate-release oral opioid is selected, and the pain is persistent or nearly so, the medication should be given every 4 hours. Once steady state has been reached, the best possible pain control for the dose will be achieved within a day (4–5 half-lives). The patient should see his or her primary physician within the next 24 to 48 hours, and he or she should be started on long-acting, continuous-release medications with breakthrough doses as needed.

Opioid-Tolerant Patients

Opioid-tolerant patients may come to the ED experiencing oligoanalgesia. They often say that their medications are no longer effective. This can be a function of physiologic tolerance, disease progression, or ineffective use of the medications (for example, taking continuous-release opioids only once per day when they were intended for 12-hour use). Opioid-tolerant patients presenting to the ED with severe pain will often need to have increases made in their baseline opioid dosing to achieve pain control.

RESPIRATORY DEPRESSION, NALOXONE, AND DOUBLE EFFECT

Emergency clinicians have a variety of concerns that make providing appropriate dosing of opioids challenging. Emergency staff, patients, and families often have concerns of addiction, misuse of the drug, and unintended outcomes, such as respiratory depression. The actual risk of respiratory depression is likely exaggerated due to the inappropriate application of animal and human models from acute pain research in opioid-naïve subjects. Respiratory depression is very unlikely in the treatment of cancer pain for patients with stable organ function.[21] The risks for respiratory depression include patients with advanced age, obesity, sleep apnea, impaired liver or renal function, side effect of sedation, and patients who achieve good pain control after long periods of poor pain control (**Box 1**).

Pain is a potent stimulus to breathe, and pharmacologic tolerance to respiratory depression develops quickly.[22] In similar doses, opioid effects are quite different in patients who are in pain and those who are not in pain. As doses increase, respiratory depression does not occur suddenly in the absence of other signs of overdose, such as lethargy and somnolence. In addition, somnolence always precedes respiratory depression. The presence of unusual somnolence provides an objective guide for safe downward adjustments (or the rare need for intervention) before the onset of respiratory depression. In addition, tolerance to the respiratory depressant effects of opioids occurs rapidly (a few days in most cases). Therefore, opioid-tolerant patients are much less susceptible to these effects.

Box 1
Risk factors for respiratory depression
Patients at increased risk for respiratory depression
• Patients who are opioid naïve
• Patients of advanced age
• Obese patients
• Patients with sleep apnea
• Patients with impaired liver or renal function
• Patients with side effect of sedation
• Patients who achieve good pain control after long periods of poor pain control

Adequate ongoing assessment and appropriate titration of opioids based on pharmacologic principles will prevent misadventures. As physiologic conditions change, opioid tolerance may change. Opioid-related respiratory depression may be an indication of a physiologic change in the patient, such as worsening renal or hepatic function, ileus, or bowel obstruction. In addition, patients who develop fever or apply heat to a transdermal patch can rapidly and dangerously elevate the drug levels. In such a situation, the removal of the transdermal patch is analogous to decontamination in an acute poisoning and should be done as quickly as possible.

Naloxone may be necessary if the cause of serious respiratory depression (rate <6/min) is an opioid. If Emergency Medical Service is called to the home of a patient for unexpected respiratory depression, an important immediate goal is to avoid an acute withdrawal state. A safe method of intervening while avoiding acute withdrawal is to dilute 0.4 mg naloxone into 10 mL of normal saline (0.04 mg/mL). Administer 0.5 mL IV every 1 to 2 minutes until respirations increase but generally not to the point of alertness. Because the effective plasma half-life is short (10–15 minutes) and because of naloxone's high affinity for lipids, the patient should be closely monitored every few minutes for recurrent drowsiness. If drowsiness recurs, dosing should be repeated (occasionally a continuous infusion is needed) as required until the patient is no longer compromised.[23]

If the primary goal of care is comfort in a patient whose only conscious experience is excruciating pain, then permissive somnolence might be acceptable. In an actively dying patient, while treating the patient's suffering with appropriate dosing of medications, the patient may finally stop breathing. With the severely impaired physiology of the actively dying patient, the addition of medications to alleviate suffering consistent with the patient's goals of care might contribute to his or her death in an unknowable way. This is the principle of "double effect," which depends entirely on the intention and actions of the treating clinician. If the clinician is using accepted medical practice to treat suffering appropriately and the patient dies, the clinician's intention has been only to alleviate symptoms. If the intention were to induce death with a dose of medication that will likely result in the patient's death, then the practice would be referred to as "physician-assisted suicide." Physician-assisted suicide is illegal in the United States except in Oregon, where its practice is carefully monitored.

OPIOID DOSING STRATEGIES

In order to provide rapid, adequate, and safe pain relief with opioids in the ED, it is important to know a patient's current medication regime. Increasing dosages by

25% to 50% per day when moderate pain persists or by 50% to 100% per day for patients with continued severe pain is considered safe practice. Understanding the pharmacokinetics of opioids, it is nevertheless prudent for patients to be observed at home during the next 24 hours (until steady state is achieved) for signs of dose-limiting toxicity. The emergency clinician should always speak with the primary care outpatient provider to ensure that the opioids can be effectively titrated and the patient receives follow-up care.

Equianalgesic dosing tables help to convert a sometimes complex array of multiple medications into a single opioid equivalent (**Table 4**). From there, a safe and effective dose for initial treatment can be implemented. When converting from one opioid to another, a helpful first step is to calculate the "oral morphine equivalent" of the patient's current opioid. The oral morphine equivalent is the dose of morphine that is of equivalent strength to the dose of the current opioid. It is usually calculated for the preceding 24-hour time period. For example, a patient who is taking 4 mg of oral hydromorphone every 4 hours is receiving 24 mg of oral hydromorphone in a 24-hour period. The oral morphine equivalent of 24 mg of oral hydromorphone is approximately 90 mg of oral morphine (24 [30/7.5] = 96, rounded down to 90). This is equivalent to 30 mg IV/subcutaneous (SQ) morphine. Accepted guidelines for the conversion of transdermal fentanyl to oral morphine are unusual in that the hourly dose of the transdermal form is equated to the daily (24 h) dose of oral morphine. For example, a 25 mcg/h transdermal fentanyl patch (which is typically maintained for 3 days) is roughly equivalent to 50 mg of oral morphine a day.[24]

OPIOID CROSS-TOLERANCE

Although patients may develop pharmacologic tolerance (a higher dose to achieve the same effect) to the opioid being used, tolerance may not be as marked relative to other opioids. Incomplete cross-tolerance is likely due to subtle differences in the molecular structure of each opioid and the way each interacts with the patient's opioid receptors. Consequently, when switching opioids, there may be differences between published equianalgesic doses of different opioids and the effective dose for a given patient. It is prudent to start with 50% to 75% of the published equianalgesic dose of the new opioid to compensate for incomplete cross-tolerance and individual variation, especially if the patient's pain is controlled. If the patient has moderate to severe pain, the dose should not be reduced as much. If the patient has had adverse effects such as sedation, the dose should be reduced even more. However, in the case of a known time-limited side effect such as nausea, the dose may be continued with a trial of treatment of the side effect.

Table 4
Equianalgesic opioid dosing table

Equianalgesic Doses of OPIOID Analgesics		
Oral/Rectal Dose (mg)	Analgesic	Parenteral Dose (mg)
100	Codeine	60
15	Hydrocodone	—
4	Hydromorphone	1
15	Morphine	5
10	Oxycodone	—

An important exception is methadone. Methadone is the only opioid shown to have a nonlinear relationship to standard opioids. For patients receiving morphine doses less than 100 mg/d, the ratio is 4:1 (morphine:methadone). However if the morphine is >1000 mg/day, the ratio is 20:1 (morphine:methadone).[23] Conversion to methadone is complex and requires expertise in the use of the drug. Expertise with administering methadone as well as close follow-up is essential for safety. Emergency clinicians should discuss any methadone dosing with a pain or palliative care consultant before adjustments to assist as well as ensure safe use.

BREAKTHROUGH DOSING

Treatment in cancer pain is guided by knowledge of the patient's current medications and dosing for baseline and breakthrough pain. Baseline pain refers to the patient's pain experience for more than 12 hours in a 24-hour period. Breakthrough pain is a moderate to severe transient increase over baseline pain.[25] Breakthrough dosing is typically 5% to 15% of the total daily dose in oral morphine equivalents every hour (Cmax). Any immediate-release opioid can be used, but care must be taken to avoid acetaminophen toxicity when combination medications are used for breakthrough dosing. Extended-release opioids should not be used for breakthrough pain, as their onset of action is too slow, and risk for cumulative toxicity is high.

BOLUS EFFECT

As the level of opioid in the bloodstream increases due to use of immediate-release preparations, some patients may experience drowsiness 1/2 to 1 hour after ingestion, when the plasma level peaks. This may be followed by pain just before the next dose is due, when the plasma level falls. The name of this syndrome is the "bolus effect," and it can best be resolved by switching to an extended-release formulation (oral, rectal, or transdermal) or a continuous parenteral infusion. This should reduce swings in the plasma concentration after each dose.[26]

ADJUVANT ANALGESICS

Adjuvant analgesics (or coanalgesics) are medications that, when added to primary analgesics, further improve pain control. They may themselves also be primary analgesics (eg, tricyclic antidepressant medications for postherpetic neuralgia). They can be added into the pain management plan at any step in the WHO ladder and are often used. Common adjuvants include the WHO step 1 medications as well as other medications used in the treatment of neuropathic pain.

Corticosteroids are potent anti-inflammatory agents that are useful in both nociceptive and neuropathic pain. Reducing inflammation and peritumor edema can be important in relieving pressure on a nerve or the spinal cord, decreasing intracranial pressure from a brain tumor, or decreasing obstruction of a hollow viscus. Corticosteroids may also be useful for bone pain, visceral pain (obstruction and/or capsular distention), anorexia, nausea, and depressed mood. At the end of life, dexamethasone is considered the corticosteroid of choice because of its minimal mineralocorticoid effects and thus its decreased tendency for salt and fluid retention. Corticosteroids may also enhance pain control through the creation of a sense of euphoria. Dexamethasone has a long half-life (>36 hours). It can be administered once a day in doses of 2 to 20 mg oral or up to 100 mg IV for acute spinal cord compression. If an agitated delirium ensues, steroid psychosis should be considered. Although proximal myopathy, oral candidiasis, bone loss, and other toxicities may occur with long-term use, this is seldom a major problem in the setting of advanced disease.

ROUTES OF ADMINISTRATION

The oral route is generally the least invasive and most convenient for administering opioids on a routine basis. However, some patients may benefit from other routes of administration if oral intake is either not possible (due to vomiting, dysphagia, or esophageal obstruction) or if it causes uncontrollable adverse effects (nausea, drowsiness, or confusion).

Enteral feeding tubes provide alternatives for bypassing gastroesophageal obstructions. They deliver the medications to the stomach or upper intestine where the medications function pharmacologically as though they had been ingested orally. Immediate-release medications or liquid medications are easily administered through feeding tubes. Long-acting preparations, however, cannot be crushed for administration. One long-acting morphine preparation Kadian has multiple time-release granules that may be removed from the capsule and administered through the feeding tube as a 24-hour, long-acting opioid. Transmucosal (buccal mucosal) administration of more concentrated, immediate-release, liquid preparations provides a similar alternative, particularly in the patient who is unable to swallow. Oral transmucosal fentanyl citrate is a formulation of fentanyl in a candy matrix on a stick that is approved for the treatment of breakthrough pain. To date, experience with this formulation and the recently released fentanyl dissolvable tablet show some usefulness for breakthrough pain, although dosing and cost are problematic. Topical anesthetic creams are currently used most commonly in pediatrics in the ED and are effective. They should be considered as well for cancer patients. Venipuncture may be intolerably painful to a patient in severe discomfort. If it is acceptable in a given situation to wait for a necessary venipuncture, topical analgesia with agents such as eutectic mixture of local anesthetics (lidocaine 2.5%/prilocaine 2.5%) or ELA-Max (4% lidocaine) should be considered.

Open wounds may also be a source of considerable pain, particularly during dressing changes or debridement. If incident pain is significant, the patient should be given medication before performing activities that cause pain. Based on Cmax for opioids, this could be 60 minutes for oral medications, 30 minutes for SQ or rectal, and 15 minutes for IV (see **Table 1**). It should be noted that these are the most conservative figures and that the Tmax of IV morphine is often quoted at 6 to 8 minutes.

In addition, topical analgesics should be considered. It is known that there are *mu* opioid receptors throughout the body, and there is some experience with the successful use of the IV form of morphine applied topically. This may be placed topically into the wound during a dressing change. Depending on the size of the wound and opioid tolerance of the patient, 4 to 20 mg of injectable morphine can be placed into an inert cream and applied directly to the wound and covered with gauze dressings.[27–29]

Transdermal patches present an effective alternative route of administration for patients who are receiving stable routine opioid dosing. These patches are currently manufactured only with fentanyl, and they perform quite differently from other extended-release formulations. Steady-state equilibrium is established between the medication in the patch, a subdermal pool that develops, and the patient's circulation. On average, best possible pain control is achieved within 1 dosing interval (ie, 3 days), with peak effect at about 24 hours. The effect usually lasts for 48 to 72 hours before the patch needs to be changed. Care must be taken to ensure that the patches are placed in an appropriate location so they absorb properly and adhere to the patient's skin. Fentanyl is highly lipophilic, so an area with adequate subcutaneous fat and no hair is the best choice. It is also important to understand that if the patch needs to be removed, the drug will continue to exert an effect for up to 12 hours after removal.

Rectal administration of prepackaged suppositories or extended-release oral morphine tablets inserted rectally behave pharmacologically like related oral preparations. This route may be very effective if oral intake is suddenly not possible, although many patients do not like this route for continuous administration.

Parenteral (IV or subcutaneous) administration using injection or infusion can be very useful in some patients. If bolus dosing is required, and IV access is either not present or difficult, the subcutaneous route is an appropriate route. The intramuscular route is not recommended. Intermittent subcutaneous injections are much less painful and just as effective. When renal function is normal, routine parenteral bolus (IV or SQ) doses should be provided every 3 hours and the dose adjusted every 12 to 24 hours once steady state is reached. If a parenteral route will be used for some time, continuous infusions may produce a more constant plasma level, reduce the risk of adverse effects, be better tolerated by the patient, and require less intervention by professional staff. Patient-controlled analgesia has been shown to be both effective and well tolerated by patients. Although intravenous infusions may be preferable when intravenous access is already established and in use for other medications, all opioids available for parenteral use may be administered subcutaneously without the discomfort associated with searching for an IV site or the risk of serious infection. Either 25- or 27-gauge needles can be used for both bolus dosing and infusions. The needles can be left in place for 7 days or more as long as there is no sign of infection or local irritation. Family members can be taught to change the needles.

Pain from tumor infiltration can cause excruciating pain, which is sometimes resistant to medications. In addition, the side effects of systemic medications used to treat pain are sometimes intolerable, even with significant supportive treatment. Anesthetic techniques such as neuraxial (epidural or intrathecal) catheter delivery of pain medication or anesthetic blocks of the involved area can sometimes help dramatically. These approaches are available through specialists in interventional pain management. This is an excellent consideration for patients with pain that is unresponsive to standard aggressive medical therapy or as an adjunct to pain management when side effects are unmanageable.

NONRECOMMENDED OPIOIDS

Not all analgesics available today are recommended. Meperidine has 2 major problems that make it undesirable, and, thus, it has been removed from many hospital formularies. Its principal metabolite, normeperidine, has no analgesic properties of its own, has a longer half-life of about 6 hours, is renally excreted, and produces significant adverse effects when it accumulates, such as tremulousness, dysphoria, myoclonus, and seizures. Additionally, meperidine is poorly absorbed orally and has a short half-life of approximately 3 hours. The routine dosing of meperidine every 3 hours for analgesia leads to unavoidable accumulation of normeperidine and exposes the patient to unnecessary risk of adverse effects, particularly if renal clearance is impaired. Consequently, meperidine is not recommended for routine dosing.

Propoxyphene is also not recommended. It has a narrow therapeutic window, standard dosing is below analgesic threshold, and dose escalation is associated with accumulation of toxic metabolites.

The mixed opioid agonist-antagonists (pentazocine, butorphanol, nalbuphine, and dezocine) cannot be used in patients who might require other opioids. If used together, competition for the opioid receptors may cause a withdrawal reaction. Furthermore, agonist-antagonists are not recommended as routine analgesics, because their dosing is limited by a ceiling effect, which precludes dose escalation, and some carry a high risk of psychotomimetic adverse effects.

OPIOID-INDUCED SIDE EFFECTS

Many people confuse opioid side effects, such as urticaria/pruritis, nausea/vomiting, constipation, drowsiness, or confusion, with allergic reactions. Although 1 or more adverse effect may present on initial dosing, they can be easily managed, and in a relatively brief period of time, patients generally develop pharmacologic tolerance to all of them (except constipation). Urticaria, pruritis, and bronchospasm could be direct opioid effects or signs of allergy. These effects are usually the result of mast cell destabilization by the opioid and subsequent histamine release. Usually, the rash and pruritus can be managed by routine administration of long-acting, nonsedating oral antihistamines while opioid dosing continues (eg, fexofenadine, 60 mg twice a day; diphenhydramine, 25 mg every 6 hours, or loratadine, 10 mg daily). True anaphylaxis, although rare with opioids, should certainly be taken very seriously, and the offending opioid should be replaced with another from a different class.

Many patients who start opioids experience nausea, with or without vomiting. It is easily anticipated and treated with antiemetics and usually disappears within a few days as tolerance develops. Young women seem to be most at risk. Dopamine-blocking agents are most often effective (eg, prochlorperazine, 10 mg before opioid and every 6 hours; haloperidol, 1 mg before opioid and every 6 hours; metoclopramide, 10 mg before opioid and every 6 hours).

PROPHYLAXIS AGAINST CONSTIPATION

Constipation secondary to opioid administration is almost universal. It is primarily the result of opioid effects on the CNS, spinal cord, and myenteric plexus of gut, which, in turn, reduce gut motor activity and increase stool transit time. The colon has more time to desiccate its contents, leaving large hard stools that are difficult to pass. Other factors, such as dehydration, poor food intake, and other medications, may make the problem worse. Tolerance to constipation may develop very slowly, if at all. It requires anticipatory and ongoing management. Dietary interventions alone (eg, increase fluid and fiber) are often insufficient. Bulk-forming agents (eg, psyllium) require substantial fluid intake and are not recommended for those with advanced disease and poor mobility.

To counteract the slowing effect of opioids, the clinician should prescribe a routine stimulant laxative (eg, senna, bisacodyl, glycerine, casanthranol, etc) and escalate the dose to effect. Although detergent laxatives or "stool softeners" (eg, docusate sodium) are usually not effective by themselves, combination stimulant/softeners (eg, senna + docusate sodium) can be useful. Prokinetic agents (eg, metoclopramide) may also counteract the opioid effect. If constipation persists, some patients will benefit from the addition of an osmotic agent, such as milk of magnesia, lactulose, or sorbitol, to increase the moisture content of the stool. Many patients have difficulty tolerating the discomfort associated with osmotic agents, so they should be considered second-line therapy when prokinetics and detergent/softener laxatives are inadequate.

When standard therapies for constipation are either inadequate or the route of administration is untenable, methylnaltrexone bromide (Relistor) may be tried. Methylnaltrexone bromide was approved in 2008 by the FDA for use in adult patients with opioid-induced constipation in advanced illness. The mechanism of action is at the gut mu receptors, where it inhibits opioid uptake. Laxation (without diminished opioid analgesia) is expected for the majority of patients within 4 hours but as early as 30 minutes, with a single dose of 0.15 mg/kg. The drug may be administered as a single subcutaneous injection every other day as needed.[30,31]

RAPID OPIOID TITRATION IN THE ED

The administration of parenteral medication in the ED, as a time-limited therapeutic trial, allows the clinician to discover what medication level a patient can safely and effectively tolerate while the patient is still in the ED. Opioid pain management in the ED can be done rapidly, safely, and effectively if analgesic principles are used. Treating the patient in the ED to establish opioid tolerance of dosing over a period of time is an important safety guard. Because maximal side effects of sleepiness, drowsiness, and respiratory depression occur at Cmax, the emergency clinician can give the patient a test dose, observe this effect, and expect a similar state in the home setting.

Oligoanalgesia in the home environment is often a reason for a patient with malignancy to seek help in the ED. The severity of pain (assessed by an appropriate pain scale) determines the approach. If the pain is assessed as severe, a rapid titration of pain medication in the ED is indicated. Adequate pain control can be achieved rapidly and safely in the ED. There are limited studies looking at rapid titration of opioids, but safety and efficacy are consistently demonstrated using standard dosing guidelines.[32–34]

If the pain is assessed as mild to moderate (<6/10), a standard history and physical examination should help determine the best intervention in the ED. The reason for oligoanalgesia may be as simple as a misunderstanding of medication dosage or interval. Communication with the primary care physician or oncologist may provide additional information to guide further interventions as well as appropriate disposition. It may make sense to provide a medication or particular dosage in the ED, by an acceptable route to the patient, to determine efficacy. By Cmax (under 90 minutes for enteral routes), if the home situation is acceptable and simple medication or dose adjustments are likely to achieve comfort, then the patient can be safely discharged with appropriate follow-up.

The following approach to the rapid treatment of cancer pain is derived from the Educating Physicians on End of Life Care-Emergency Medicine[35] curriculum:

Step 1: Assess

- Is this pain, despite its intensity, familiar in character to the patient, or is this a new pain?
- Is this likely related to the cancer or something unrelated?
- Is this progressive baseline pain (>12/24 h) or breakthrough pain?
- What medication and dosage has the patient taken for pain control in the past 24 to 48 hours? What is the response (degree of pain relief and duration of effect) to a given dose of each medication? When was the last dose?
- If severe (>7/10), initiate treatment (step 2):
- If mild to moderate pain (and when severe pain is better controlled):
  - Is the patient taking home medications appropriately?
  - Is the pain expected to be more opioid responsive (nociceptive) or less opioid responsive (neuropathic)?
  - Are appropriate adjuvant therapies being used?
  - Are there serious diagnostic concerns to be addressed emergently within the patient's goals of care?

Step 2: Treat

- Severe pain (>7/10): The optimal route for rapid titration of severe pain is IV (if a port or first-attempt peripheral vein is accessible) or SQ.
  - Opioid naïve: Administer parenteral morphine equivalent to 0.1 mg/kg (less if in a high-risk group).
  - Opioid tolerant: Administer 5% of the patient's total previous 24-hour parenteral morphine equivalents, minimum 0.1 mg/kg (less if patient is in a high-risk group).
- Mild to moderate pain: Consider best route and choice of medication based on assessment and goals of care.

Step 3: Reassess

- Perform pain severity assessment at Cmax (15 minutes after completion of intravenous pyelogram or intravenous piggyback dose, 30 minutes after SQ injection, 60–90 minutes after enteral route).
- Are there unwanted side effects (somnolence, confusion)?

Step 4: Achieve Adequate Pain Control

- Persistent severe pain (>7/10) without unmanageable side effects: Double the opioid dose.
- Some response but inadequate relief of pain (<50% improvement): Repeat same opioid dose.

Repeat steps 3 and 4 until pain is controlled or unwanted side effects occur, or limit further escalation.

Step 5: Determine Plan for Disposition, Discharge Instructions, and Follow-up

- Patients who cannot be reasonably controlled over a period of dose escalation and observation in the ED should be considered for hospital admission.
- The choice of a long-acting regimen depends on the patient's previous opioid use, the ability to swallow, the allergy profile, and what has been tolerated in the past. With the exception of methadone (which may have some activity in neuropathic pain), there is no commonly accepted advantage of any particular long-acting opioid. Because of its complicated dosing, methadone should not be initiated or titrated from the ED without consultation from the patient's primary care physician or a specialist in pain or palliative medicine.
- After achieving adequate pain control with the increase in long-acting opioids accompanied by appropriate breakthrough dosing, discharge instructions and follow-up with the oncologist or primary physician should be arranged.

SUMMARY

Patients and families struggling with cancer fear pain more than any other physical symptom. A basic understanding of pain assessment, opioid pharmacology, equianalgesic conversions, rationale for opioid dose escalations, and management of side effects can enhance a clinician's ability not only to effectively manage pain but also to enhance patient safety.

REFERENCES

1. van den Beuken-van Everdingen MH, de Rijke JM, Kessels AG, et al. Prevalence of pain in patients with cancer: a systematic review of the past 40 years. Ann Oncol 2007;18(9):1437–49.
2. Ventafridda VOE, Caraceni A. A retrospective study on the use of oral morphine in cancer pain. J Pain Symptom Manage 1987;2:77–82.
3. Walker VA, Hoskin PJ, Hanks GW, et al. Evaluation of WHO analgesic guidelines for cancer pain in a hospital-based palliative care unit. J Pain Symptom Manage 1988;3:145–9.
4. Goisis A, Gorini M, Ratti R, et al. Application of a WHO protocol on medical therapy for oncologic pain in an internal medicine hospital. Tumori 1989;75:470–2.
5. Caraceni A, Martini C, Zecca E, et al. Breakthrough pain characteristics and syndromes in patients with cancer pain. An international survey. Pa Med 2004; 18:177–83.
6. Zech DF, Grond S, Lynch J, et al. Validation of World Health Organization guidelines for cancer pain relief: a 10-year prospective study. Pain 1995;63:65–76.
7. Mercadante S. Pain treatment and outcomes for patients with advanced cancer who receive follow-up care at home. Cancer 1999;85:1849–58.
8. Moryl N, Coyle N, Foley KM. Managing an acute pain crisis in a patient with advanced cancer: "this is as much of a crisis as a code". JAMA 2008;299(12): 1457–67.
9. Todd KH. Pain assessment instruments for use in the emergency department. Emerg Med Clin North Am 2005;23:285–95.
10. Ramer L, Richardson JL, Cohen MZ, et al. Multimeasure pain assessment in an ethnically diverse group of patients with cancer. J Transcult Nurs 1999;10: 94–101.
11. DeWaters T, Faut-Callahan M, McCann JJ, et al. Comparison of self-reported pain and the PAINAD scale in hospitalized cognitively impaired and intact older adults after hip fracture surgery. Orthop Nurs 2008;27(1):28–30.
12. Zwakhalen SM, hamers JP, Berger MP. The psychometric quality and clinical usefulness of three pain assessment tools for elderly people with dementia. Pain 2006;126(1–3):210–20.
13. Foley KM. Acute and chronic cancer pain syndromes. In: Doyle D, Hanks G, Cherny K, et al, editors. Oxford textbook of palliative medicine. New York: Oxford University Press; 2004. p. 298–316.
14. Bruera E, Neumann CM, Gagnon B, et al. Edmonton Regional Palliative Care Program: impact on patterns of terminal cancer care. CMAJ 1999;161(3):290–3.
15. Breitbart W, Chochinov HM, Passik SD. Psychiatric symptoms in palliative medicine. In: Doyle D, Hanks G, Cherny K, et al, editors. Oxford textbook of palliative medicine. New York: Oxford University Press; 2004. p. 746–71.
16. Casarett D, Pickard A, Bailey FA, et al. "Do palliative consultations improve patient outcomes?" J Am Geriatr Soc 2008;56(4):593–9.
17. Bruhlmann P, Florent dV, Dreiser, et al. Short-term treatment with topical diclofenac epolamine plaster in patients with symptomatic knee osteoarthritis: pooled analysis of two randomised clinical studies. Curr Med Res Opin 2006;22(12):2429–38.
18. Dean M. Opioids in renal failure and dialysis patients. J Pain Symptom Manage 2004;28(5):497–504.
19. Broadbent A, Khor K, Heaney A. Palliation and chronic renal failure: opioid and other palliative medications – dosage guidelines. Progr Palliat Care 2003;11(4): 183–90.

20. Murphy EJ. Acute pain management pharmacology for the patient with concurrent renal or hepatic disease. Anaesth Intensive Care 2005;33(3):311–22.

21. Estfan B, Mahmoud F, Shaheen P, et al. Respiratory function during parenteral opioid titration for cancer pain. Pa Med 2007;21(2):81–6.

22. Smith LH. Opioid safety: is your patient at risk for respiratory depression? Clin J Oncol Nurs 2007;11(2):293–6.

23. Abrams JL. Pharmacological management of cancer pain. A physician's guide to pain and symptom management in cancer patients. Baltimore (MD): The Johns Hopkins University Press; 2005. p. 197–9, 242.

24. Skaer TL. Practice guidelines for transdermal opioids in malignant pain. Drugs 2004;64(23):2629–38.

25. Portenoy RK, Hagen NA. "Breakthrough pain: definition, prevalence and characteristics". Pain Headache 1990;41:273–82.

26. Cherny N, Ripamonti C, Pereira J, et al. Expert Working Group of the European Association of Palliative Care Network. Strategies to manage the adverse effects of oral morphine: an evidence-based report. J Clin Oncol 2001;19(9):2542–54.

27. Krajnik M, Zylicz Z, Finlay I, et al. Potential uses of topical opioids in palliative care—report of 6 cases. Pain 1999;80(1–2):121–5.

28. Zeppetella G, Paul J, Ribeiro MDC. Analgesic efficacy of morphine applied topically to painful ulcers. J Pain Symptom Manage 2003;25:555–8.

29. Zeppetella G, Ribeiro MDC. Morphine in Intrasite gel applied topically to painful ulcers. J Pain Symptom Manage 2005;29:118–9.

30. Portenoy RK, Thomas J, Boatwright MLM, et al. Subcutaneous methylnaltrexone for the treatment of opioid-induced constipation in patients with advanced illness: a double-blind, randomized, parallel group, dose-ranging study. J Pain Symptom Manage 2008;35:458–68.

31. Thomas J, Karver S, Cooney GA, et al. Methylnaltrexone for opioid-induced constipation in advanced illness. N Engl J Med 2008;358:2332–43.

32. Mercadante S, Villari P, Ferrera P, et al. "Rapid titration with intravenous morphine for severe cancer pain and immediate oral conversion". Cancer 2002;95(1):203–8.

33. Soares LGL, Martins M, Uchoa R. Intravenous fentanyl for cancer pain: a "Fast Titration" protocol for the emergency room". J Pain Symptom Manage 2003;26(3):876–81.

34. Hagen NA, Elwood T, Ernst S. "Cancer pain emergencies: a protocol for management". J Pain Symptom Manage 1997;14(1):45–50.

35. The EPEC Project. Module 12: Malignant Pain. In: Emanuel LL, Quest TE, editors. The education in palliative and end-of-life care-emergency medicine (EPEC-EM) trainer's guide. Chicago (IL): Northwestern University; 2008.

Optimal Management of Malignant Epidural Spinal Cord Compression

Hai Sun, MD, PhD, Andrew N. Nemecek, MD*

KEYWORDS

- Epidural • Malignant • Management • Neoplasm
- Spinal cord compression

Malignant epidural spinal cord compression (MESCC) is a common complication in patients with advanced neoplasm. This disease occurs when cancer metastasizes to the spine or epidural space and compresses the spinal cord.[1] Patients usually present with acute deterioration of neurologic functions such as inability to ambulate due to the mass effect of the metastatic diseases on the spinal cord. It is of paramount importance that the emergency department (ED) physician appreciate that MESCC is considered a treatable medical emergency, and that prompt management requires swift decision making with the collaboration of specialists such as oncologists, imaging and pathology specialists, and spine surgeons to avoid further deterioration of the patient's neurologic functions.[1–5] The management strategy for MESCC has evolved over the years, in part due to technological advancements in spinal instrumentation. Herein the authors present a primer for the ED team on the epidemiology, pathophysiology, and clinical presentation of MESCC, describe the role of medical and surgical approaches in managing this disease, and, based on recent data, recommend guidelines for use in clinical practice.

EPIDEMIOLOGY

In the United States, approximately 500,000 deaths are attributable to metastatic disease every year. Of all osseous sites, the spinal column is the most common location for metastatic deposits.[6] Almost all major types of systemic cancer can metastasize to the spinal column. Evidence suggests that 2.5% to 5.0% of patients with terminal cancers have spinal involvement within the last 2 years of illness, and MESCC occurs in up to 40% of patients who have pre-existing nonspinal metastases.[3–5] The

Department of Neurological Surgery, CH8N, Oregon Health and Science University, 3303 SW Bond Avenue, Portland, OR 97239, USA
* Corresponding author.
E-mail address: nemeceka@ohsu.edu (A.N. Nemecek).

Emerg Med Clin N Am 27 (2009) 195–208
doi:10.1016/j.emc.2009.02.001
0733-8627/09/$ – see front matter © 2009 Elsevier Inc. All rights reserved.

incidence of MESCC varies by primary disease site and patient age. In adults, the most common primary tumor sites leading to MESCC are the prostate, breast, and lung, each accounting for 15% to 20% of all cases. Non-Hodgkin lymphoma, renal cell carcinoma, and multiple myeloma account for 5% to 10%, and the remainder of cases are due to colorectal sarcomas and other unknown primary tumors.[2] In the pediatric population, neuroblastoma, Ewing sarcoma, Wilms tumor, lymphoma, and soft-tissue and bone sarcoma are the most common types that lead to spinal cord compression.[7,8] The most common level of MESCC involvement is the thoracic spine (60%–78%), followed by the lumbar (16%–33%) and cervical spine (4%–15%); multiple levels are involved in up to 50% of patients.[9,10]

PATHOPHYSIOLOGY

The most common way by which a primary malignancy spreads to the spinal column is through direct arterial embolization of tumor cells. Classically, it is believed that the valveless venous system in the spine (Batson's plexus) may facilitate the hematogenous spread of the primary tumor to the spinal column.[11] Recent evidence from animals suggests that arterial embolization may be a more important mechanism for metastasis.[12] This seeding of tumor cells results in an expansive mass in the vertebral body. Compression of the epidural space can be caused by the continued growth and expansion of the mass itself or from retropulsion of bony fragments following collapse of a vertebral body weakened by tumor (**Fig. 1**). Additionally, some tumors, especially lymphoma and neuroblastoma, can reach the epidural space by the direct growth of the paravertebral tumor into the spinal canal through an intervertebral foramen.[9] Intramedullary, subdural or lepomeningeal metastases are rarely encountered causes of MESCC.[12]

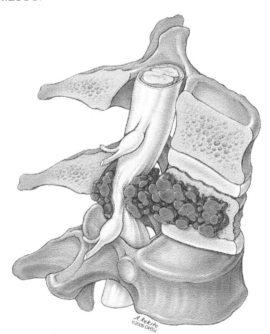

Fig. 1. Metastatic tumor invading the thoracic vertebral body causing circumferential epidural compression of the spinal cord. (*Courtesy of* OHSU Neurological Surgery, Portland, OR; with permission.)

Animal studies and intraoperative observations have demonstrated that damage to the functional integrity of the spinal cord caused by MESCC is largely due to vascular compromise. First, the tumor mass or bony fragment impinges on the venous plexus surrounding the cord, which results in cord edema. The increased edema causes increased pressure on small arterioles, which leads to diminished capillary blood flow. Disruption of blood flow to the cord leads to white matter ischemia and, with prolonged compression, may eventually cause cord infarction.[13] Production of vascular endothelial growth factor (VEGF) is also associated with spinal cord hypoxia. It has been proposed that steroid efficacy in the treatment of acute MESCC is at least partly due to down-regulation of VEGF expression.[12,14]

Another important mechanism by which metastatic tumors can harm the spinal cord is destabilization of the spinal column. Tumor invasion of the bony spine can lead to failure of the spinal column in the same way as a traumatic injury. Denis proposed a 3-column model for the evaluation of spine stability.[15] In this model (**Fig. 2**), the anterior column is composed of the anterior longitudinal ligament, the anterior annulus, and the anterior portion of the vertebral body. The middle column includes the posterior longitudinal ligament, the posterior annulus, and the posterior portion of the vertebral body. The posterior column includes those spinal structures that are posterior to the posterior longitudinal ligament. Disruption of 2 or 3 columns creates an unstable spine. It has been recognized that it is more common for a malignant lesion to involve the vertebral body and cause it to collapse. Findlay reported, in a small series, that more than half of patients with MESCC had a collapsed vertebral body.[16] Collapse often involved the anterior and middle columns, hence spinal instability.

CLINICAL PRESENTATION

Pretreatment neurologic status is by far the most important predictor of function after treatment.[2,4,6] Therefore, it is highly desirable to diagnose MESCC before the patient develops any neurologic deficits. Most patients with MESCC have a known cancer diagnosis, emphasizing the importance of providing ED personnel with ready access to the prior medical records.

Pain is by far the most common presenting symptom of MESCC, occurring in approximately 83% to 95% of patients. Back pain caused by MESCC can take several forms and local and quality can vary. Initially, pain can be localized and confined to the

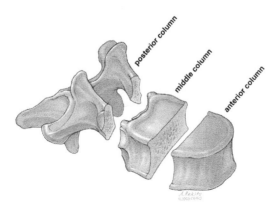

Fig. 2. Denis' 3-column model of spinal stability. Disruption of 2 or 3 columns may lead to structural instability. (*Courtesy of* OHSU Neurological Surgery, Portland, OR; with permission.)

region of spinal metastases, as the tumor stretches the periosteum or invades adjacent soft tissues. Radicular pain is also common among patients with MESCC and may occur when the tumor mass compresses or invades the nerve roots. Pain is usually worse at night when the patient is recumbent due to lengthening of the spine, or with Valsalva maneuver. A more ominous type of pain is mechanical back pain, which is made worse by movement and partially relieved with rest, may suggest spinal instability caused by vertebral body collapse.[1] This can be a harbinger of subsequent neurologic deterioration. Hence the ED triage team must maintain equipoise when evaluating patients with the common complaint of back pain.

Motor deficit is the second most common symptom of MESCC (60%–85%), followed by sensory deficits (40%–80%). Patient complaints related to these symptoms are often vague. Weakness is frequently described as clumsiness or heaviness which can progress to paralysis. Motor deficit can involve upper and lower motor neurons. Upper motor neuron weakness is more likely to be symmetric, whereas lower motor neuron weakness is often asymmetric and affects the distal end of limbs first.[17,18] Loss of ability to ambulate is usually due to weakness. Sensory deficits rarely occur before motor deficits or pain, and they usually begin distally and ascend as the disease advances.[17,18] Increased susceptibility to falling can indicate the progression of motor and sensory deficits. Autonomic/sphincter dysfunction is typically a later finding (40%–60%).[9,17,19,20] Among elderly patients, urinary retention is a more reliable sign of autonomic sphincter dysfunction than urinary incontinence. Sphincter dysfunction is a poor prognostic indicator for preservation or improvement of ambulatory status.[1]

DIAGNOSIS

A diagnosis of MESCC begins with obtaining a medical history and performing an appropriately focused general physical examination that is coupled with a comprehensive central nervous system (CNS) examination in patients suspected of having MESCC. New onset of back pain or neurologic symptoms such as symmetric weakness or paresthesia in a patient with known cancer should prompt further workup for MESCC. Imaging of the entire spine should be performed on any patient suspected of having MESCC not only to define the diagnosis but also to aid surgical or radiotherapy treatment planning. Magnetic resonance (MR) imaging is currently the gold standard imaging modal for assessing spinal metastatic disease. It is sensitive (93%) and specific (97%) for detection of MESCC[10,11] and because multiple levels are frequently involved, imaging of the entire spine is highly recommended.[21] Conventional computed tomography myelography techniques, with or without MR imaging are used if a patient cannot have MR imaging due to metallic implants.

Other imaging modalities are less useful than MR imaging. Plain films have insufficient sensitivity and specificity to make a diagnosis and they should not be performed; delaying MR imaging should be avoided.[22,23] Radionuclide bone scans and positron emission tomography can detect MESCC but they are not as accurate as MR imaging due to lower resolutions.

MANAGEMENT

Patients with MESCC are usually affected by widespread cancer. Large retrospective studies have reported the median survival time for a patient with MESCC as 3 to 6 months.[4,7] Treatment of spinal metastatic diseases including MESCC is mainly palliative. The goals are to control pain, avoid complications, and preserve neurologic function.

Corticosteroids

Corticosteroids are believed to delay neurologic deterioration by decreasing spinal cord edema and may also have an oncolytic effect on certain tumors, such as lymphoma and multiple myeloma.

As alluded to earlier, the efficacy of corticosteroids in managing patients with MESCC can partially be explained by a role in reduction of hypoxic spinal tissue VEGF expression. In a randomized trial, patients with MESCC were assigned to the treatment arm of a 96-mg intravenous (IV) bolus of dexamethasone followed by 96 mg/d orally for 3 days and a 10-day taper, versus no corticosteroids before radiotherapy. In the group treated with dexamethasone and radiation, ambulatory rates were higher than the group treated with radiation alone at 3 months and 6 months ($P<.05$).[24]

Although the efficacy of corticosteroids in delaying neurologic deterioration has been proven through these clinical data, the optimal loading and maintenance doses of corticosteroids have not been determined. Studies in animals have found a positive dose-dependent association of dexamethasone's effect in reducing cord edema, which reaches a maximum effect at approximately 100 mg/kg. Vecht and colleagues,[25] in the only randomized trial examining corticosteroid loading dose, reported no difference between an intravenous dexamethasone loading dose of 10 mg versus 100 mg with respect to pain reduction, ambulation, or bladder function. In this trial, the maintenance dose for all patients was 16 mg of oral dexamethasone per day.

Currently, due to lack of consensus, there are 2 widely used dosing regimens for steroids: a high dose (100 mg loading dose, followed by 96 mg/d) and a moderate dose (10 mg loading dose, followed by 16 mg/d). Some physicians advocate using motor symptoms to titrate the steroid dosage; that is, patients with rapidly progressive motor symptoms such as loss of ability to ambulate receive a high dose, whereas patients with minimal or nonprogressive weakness are treated with moderate doses.

Radiation

Palliative radiation therapy has been the standard care for patients with MESCC since the 1950s. The efficacy of radiotherapy in the preservation or improvement of neurologic function in patients with MESCC has been reported in numerous retrospective studies.[4,7,9,26–30] Given a lack of equipoise regarding the efficacy of radiation therapy, a prospective, randomized controlled trial comparing radiation to no radiation would not be ethical. Despite general acceptance of the effectiveness of radiotherapy, the optimal dose and treatment regimen remains controversial. In conventional external-beam fractionated radiotherapy, the proximity of the spinal cord limits the dose that can be delivered. Various dose schedules have been tried for pain relief and reversal of compression. In a systematic review of various dose schedules, Sze and colleagues[31] found no differences in pain relief between single fraction and multifraction radiotherapy. In 1 randomized study, Maranzono and colleagues,[29] reported that a hypofractionation schedule resulted in no difference in back pain relief, maintenance of ambulation, and good bladder function rates among patients with MESCC receiving radiotherapy. In a retrospective study, post-treatment ambulatory rate and motor function improvement were not shown to be affected by the initial dose and number of fractions, but the rate of in-field recurrence was lower with protracted schedules.[30] Because fractionation helps lower the risk of spinal cord injury, the recommendation based on these studies is to give a single fraction of 8 Gy to MESCC patients with limited survival expectations and 3 Gy in 10 fractions to all other patients.

Most radiation oncologists adhere to typical schedules of 2.5 to 3.6 Gy delivered in 10 to 15 fractions.

Known predictors of outcome with radiation therapy are: (1) extent of functional limitation at the start of radiation; (2) tumor type; and (3) rapidity of onset of neurologic deficits. For example, 80% to 100% of patients who are still ambulatory when they begin radiation therapy maintain their ability to walk, whereas only one third of patients who are not mobile before treatment regain the ability to walk.[7,30] Primary tumors most sensitive to radiation are lymphoma and seminomatous germ-cell tumor. Most solid tumors, such as breast, prostate, and lung cancers, are considered intermediately radiosensitive. Melanoma, osteosarcoma, and renal cell carcinoma are usually considered to be radioresistant.[32] Although patients with radioresistant tumors may still experience substantial palliation with radiation, the chance of major functional recovery or long-term response to radiation is much less than that for patients with radiosensitive tumors.[7,30] Patients who rapidly develop neurologic deficits are less likely to improve than those who develop deficits more gradually. This may reflect the fact that patients with sudden onset of paralysis have actually suffered an infarction of the spinal cord itself, which is not likely to improve even with relief of the compression. A much weaker predictor of outcome is the extent of subarachnoid block observed on MR imaging; an epidural metastasis that causes minor compression should have a better outcome than a large mass that encircles and deforms the spinal cord, and obliterates the subarachnoid space.[7]

Surgical Treatment

The role of surgical decompression in the management of patients with MESCC has evolved over the years. Historically, radiation alone was the standard treatment for MESCC, largely due to an early study comparing the efficacy of laminectomy followed by radiotherapy with that of radiotherapy alone; no difference in outcome or survival was reported.[9,33] Surgery at that time was a laminectomy that usually did not address the primary site of compression. Laminectomy decompressed the spinal canal and spinal cord but had only been proven to be effective if compression was posterior. As mentioned earlier, MESCC more commonly involves the anterior elements of the spinal column, such as the vertebral body.[16] In the setting of anterior spinal compression, a laminectomy is insufficient to achieve decompression; furthermore, it may lead to loss of spinal stability if the posterior column is disrupted, resulting in neurologic deterioration after surgery. Therefore, this procedure should be reserved for the removal of posterior lesions.

In the 1980s, with the advancement of surgical techniques and spinal instrumentation, it became possible to decompress the spinal cord circumferentially, and reconstruct and immediately stabilize the spine. This procedure can be done by combining an anterior approach, for example, thoracotomy, with a posterior approach, for example, laminectomy and fixation. For the thoracic spine, the most common location of MESCC, a single posterolateral approach can be used. This procedure involves removing anterior compressive lesions, reconstructing the anterior and middle columns of the spine, and restoring the stability of the posterior columns using segmental fixation with pedicle screws and rods (**Figs. 3–6**). A sagittal MR image showing epidural compression of the thoracic spinal cord in a 50-year-old patient with metastatic melanoma and postoperative radiographs of the same patient showing spinal hardware after decompression and stabilization are presented in **Fig. 7**. The advantage of surgical treatment over radiotherapy alone has been suggested in several uncontrolled surgical series.[34–45] In a meta-analysis, Klimo and colleagues[28] reviewed data from 24 surgical articles (999 patients) and 4 radiation

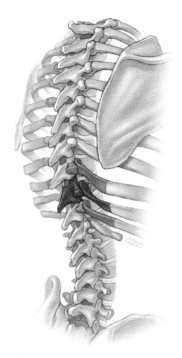

Fig. 3. Area of bony resection for posterolateral approach to anterior and posterior thoracic spinal lesions. (*Courtesy of* OHSU Neurological Surgery, Portland, OR; with permission.)

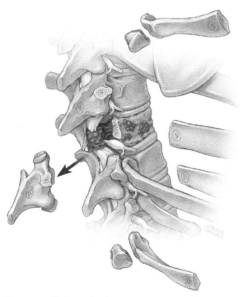

Fig. 4. Posterolateral approach to spinal metastases. T10 lamina, pedicle, and transverse process are removed. T9 and T10 ribs are removed to a distance of 10 cm from the spine, allowing extrapleural dissection and access to the ventral vertebral body. (*Courtesy of* OHSU Neurological Surgery, Portland, OR; with permission.)

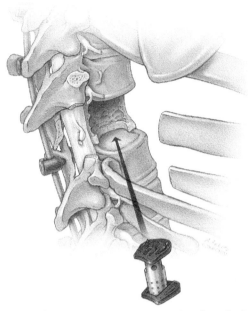

Fig. 5. Pedicle screws and a connecting rod have been placed on the left side to stabilize the spine. The vertebral body and tumor have been resected using a right posterolateral approach, and an expandable titanium cage is then placed into the resection cavity again through a right posterolateral approach, reaching around and under the spinal cord to implant the cage. (*Courtesy of* OHSU Neurological Surgery, Portland, OR; with permission.)

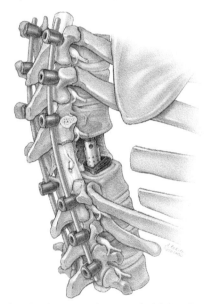

Fig. 6. Final construct. The titanium cage is expanded into place, and screws and rods are placed down the right side. The spine has now been completely decompressed and reconstructed circumferentially though a single posterolateral approach. (*Courtesy of* OHSU Neurological Surgery, Portland, OR; with permission.)

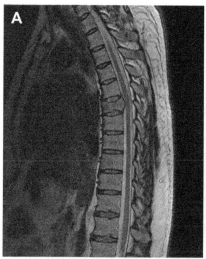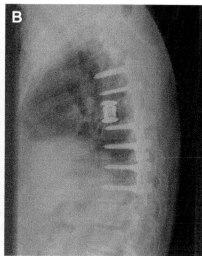

Fig. 7. Illustrative case. Sagittal MR image showing epidural compression of the thoracic spinal cord in a 50-year-old patient with metastatic melanoma (A); postoperative radiographs of the same patient showing spinal hardware after decompression and stabilization (B). (*Courtesy of* OHSU Neurological Surgery, Portland, OR; with permission.)

articles (543 patients), and reported that surgery followed by radiation leads to higher overall ambulatory success rates than radiation alone (85% vs 64%, *P*<.001).

In 2005, Patchell and colleagues[46] published the first randomized trial that compared direct decompressive and reconstructive surgery followed by postoperative radiotherapy with radiotherapy alone. The study included patients with a known cancer diagnosis, who became symptomatic from MESCC (also demonstrated with MR imaging). All patients in the study were given a loading dose of 100 mg of dexamethasone and then a maintenance dose of 24 mg every 6 hours before being randomly assigned to 1 of the 2 treatment groups. Patients in the radiotherapy alone group received 30 Gy (10 doses of 3 Gy) and the first dose of radiation began within 24 hours of enrollment in the study. Patients in the surgery followed by radiotherapy group were operated on within 24 hours of enrollment in the study and then received radiation within 2 weeks after the surgery. Surgery was performed with the intent of removing as much tumor as possible, and providing immediate decompression and stabilization of the spinal column with the necessary hardware. The primary endpoint of the study was the ability to ambulate after treatment and secondary endpoints included post-treatment continence rates, length of time patients maintained muscle strength, and functional status and survival time. The original study design called for a sample size of 200 patients but the study was stopped early after an interim analysis. One-hundred and one patients were ultimately enrolled in the study over a 10-year period. The percentage of patients able to walk after treatment was significantly (*P* = .001) higher in the surgical group (84%) than in the radiotherapy group (57%). Patients treated with surgery also retained the ability to walk significantly longer than those with radiotherapy alone (median 122 days vs 13 days, *P*<.003). Thirty-two patients (16 in each treatment group) enrolled in the study were unable to walk; a significantly greater proportion of patients in the surgery group regained the ability to walk than patients in the radiation alone group (62% vs 19%, *P* = .01). The need for corticosteroids and opioid analgesics was significantly lower in the surgical group, and muscle strength and functional status were also maintained significantly longer in patients treated with surgery. Survival times were also significantly longer in the surgery group (median, 126 days vs 100 days, $P = .033$). This landmark study confirmed the advantage of a surgical approach in treating MESCC: immediate relief of spinal compression, and stabilization of a diseased and weakened vertebral column.[46] Although this randomized trial clearly established the effectiveness of complex spinal surgery in treating MESCC, the study inclusion criteria prevents the application of data to all patients with this condition. Patients with radiosensitive tumors, neurologic deficits longer than 48 hours, multiple spinal lesions, a mass that compressed only cauda equina or spinal root, and previous radiation treatment were excluded from the study. Given the study limitations, it is incorrect to assume that all patients with MESCC would benefit from surgical treatments. One must consider whether a given patient is medically suitable for surgery. Moreover, if it is unlikely that the patient will live beyond a few weeks or months due to their oncologic disease, it may not be reasonable to perform a surgical procedure that may require several weeks of hospitalization for recovery.

Among the indications for surgical intervention, patient life expectancy is the most difficult to estimate, and the judgment and experience of specialists has been found to be inaccurate.[47–49] Several schemes and a model have been developed to predict the survival of a patient affected by MESCC, however, the predictive values of these systems have been unsatisfactory.[47,48,50,51] In general, many experts believe that factors such as the patient's functional status, the number of metastases in the vertebral body, metastases to the major internal organs (lungs, liver, kidneys, and brain), and the type of primary tumor, all have direct impact on survival. However, an estimate of how these factors influence survival rates remains qualitative.

It is commonly accepted that the goal of direct decompressive surgery is to preserve or recover ambulatory function. In several studies, preoperative ambulatory ability was found to be strongly associated with postoperative ambulation, namely patients who were able to walk before the surgery were likely to retain the ability to walk.[6,34,35,46,52–55] These data suggest that early surgical intervention may benefit patients before ambulatory function begins to decline.

Emerging Treatment Options

Spinal stereotactic radiosurgery (SRS) and other emerging forms of radiotherapy, such as intensity-modulated radiotherapy, allow radiation to be more accurately delivered to the target while minimizing the amount delivered to normal issues. Conventional radiotherapy is typically administered in 10 to 15 fractions with a total radiation dose of 25 to 40 Gy.[30] Stereotactic localization enables multiple radiation beams to converge on the lesion of interest at a high dose, while limiting the exposure of normal tissue. As a result, SRS can be administered in 1 or 2 sessions on an outpatient basis with total dose ranges of 8 to18 Gy. Degen and colleagues,[56] using the CyberKnife frameless robotic radiosurgery system to treat 58 spinal metastatic lesions, reported a significant improvement in pain. Of patients who presented with a neurologic deficit, less than one third improved. The study also demonstrated that SRS produced only mild side effects, maintaining quality of life for the patients. There is a need to test the effectiveness of spinal SRS versus surgery and radiotherapy in the setting of acute MESCC. Shortcomings of SRS include an inability to address the issue of spinal instability and delivery of radiation to large lesions.

Percutaneous vertebroplasty and kyphoplasty have received considerable attention due to their minimal invasiveness. There has been some evidence that these procedures can lead to marked pain relief in patients with intractable pain secondary to pathologic vertebral body fractures.[57] It is to be hoped that these techniques can provide the same pain relief for patients with MESCC when combined with radiotherapy. In an attempt to identify factors predicting ambulatory status after decompressive surgery, Chaichana and colleagues[52] reported that the presence of a pathologic compression fracture on preoperative images was independently associated with postoperative loss of ambulation. This finding prompted the investigators to advocate prompt treatment of metastatic disease before the onset of compression fractures using techniques such as vertebroplasty and kyphoplasty. These treatment options can only be considered if the patient is free of neurologic signs and symptoms caused by vertebral body collapse or tumor extension. The presence of these signs and symptoms is currently considered a relative contraindication for vertebroplasty and kyphoplasty.

Chemotherapy is rarely used in acute management of MESCC because, even with chemosensitive tumors, the response is too slow and unpredictable for it to be effective. In the case of chemosensitive tumors, chemotherapy may be used in conjunction with radiotherapy. Chemotherapy may also be given if a patient who has undergone radiotherapy for cord compression has recurrence and is no longer a candidate for further surgery or radiation.[58,59]

SUMMARY

The management of malignant spinal cord compression has evolved with advances in surgical techniques, chemotherapeutics, and radiation delivery. A growing body of evidence has emerged; including Level I data from a prospective, randomized controlled trial, demonstrating the efficacy of combining surgery with radiation in the treatment of spinal metastases. Clearly, a multidisciplinary approach is necessary to facilitate the management of this oncologic emergency. This approach involves spine surgeons, radiation, and medical oncologists, as well as imaging and pathology specialists. Moreover, the emergency medicine physician is often the "front door" to this multidisciplinary approach. Particularly in cases of previously undiagnosed cancer, it is often the emergency physician who makes the diagnosis and engages the appropriate specialists.

Patients with malignancy who present with new onset of neurologic signs and symptoms should undergo emergent evaluation including MR imaging of the entire spine. If MESCC is diagnosed, patients should receive an intravenous loading dose of 10 mg dexamethasone followed by a maintenance dose of 4 to 6 mg (intravenous or oral) every 6 to 8 hours. Simultaneously, the spine surgery and oncology teams should be immediately consulted. If indicated, patients should undergo maximal tumor resection and stabilization, followed by postoperative radiotherapy administered in 10 to 15 fractions with a total radiation dose of 25 to 40 Gy. In patients for whom surgery is contraindicated, palliative radiotherapy still remains the standard of care. Emerging treatment options such as stereotactic radiosurgery and vertebroplasty may be able to provide some symptomatic relief for patients who cannot undergo surgery.

ACKNOWLEDGMENTS

The authors would like to express their appreciation and thanks to Shirley McCartney, PhD, for editorial assistance, and Andy Rekito, MS, for assistance with digital illustrations.

REFERENCES

1. Cole JS, Patchell RA. Metastatic epidural spinal cord compression. Lancet Neurol 2008;7:459–66.
2. Bach F, Larsen BH, Rohde K, et al. Metastatic spinal cord compression. Occurrence, symptoms, clinical presentations and prognosis in 398 patients with spinal cord compression. Acta Neurochir 1990;107:37–43.
3. Byrne TN. Spinal cord compression from epidural metastases [see comment]. N Engl J Med 1992;327:614–9.
4. Loblaw DA, Laperriere NJ, Mackillop WJ. A population-based study of malignant spinal cord compression in Ontario. Clin Oncol (R Coll Radiol) 2003;15:211–7.
5. Quinn JA, DeAngelis LM. Neurologic emergencies in the cancer patient. Semin Oncol 2000;27:311–21.
6. Aaron AD. The management of cancer metastatic to bone. JAMA 1994;272:1206–9.
7. Helweg-Larsen S, Sorensen PS, Kreiner S. Prognostic factors in metastatic spinal cord compression: a prospective study using multivariate analysis of variables influencing survival and gait function in 153 patients. Int J Radiat Oncol Biol Phys 2000;46:1163–9.
8. Raffel C, Neave VC, Lavine S, et al. Treatment of spinal cord compression by epidural malignancy in childhood. Neurosurgery 1991;28:349–52.
9. Gilbert RW, Kim JH, Posner JB. Epidural spinal cord compression from metastatic tumor: diagnosis and treatment. Ann Neurol 1978;3:40–51.
10. Schiff D, O'Neill BP, Wang CH, et al. Neuroimaging and treatment implications of patients with multiple epidural spinal metastases. Cancer 1998;83:1593–601.
11. Li KC, Poon PY. Sensitivity and specificity of MRI in detecting malignant spinal cord compression and in distinguishing malignant from benign compression fractures of vertebrae. Magn Reson Imaging 1988;6:547–56.
12. Arguello F, Baggs RB, Duerst RE, et al. Pathogenesis of vertebral metastasis and epidural spinal cord compression. Cancer 1990;65:98–106.
13. Siegal T. Spinal cord compression: from laboratory to clinic. Eur J Cancer 1995; 31A:1748–53.
14. Benton RL, Whittemore SR. VEGF165 therapy exacerbates secondary damage following spinal cord injury. Neurochem Res 2003;28:1693–703.
15. Denis F. The three column spine and its significance in the classification of acute thoracolumbar spinal injuries. Spine 1983;8:817–31.
16. Findlay GF. The role of vertebral body collapse in the management of malignant spinal cord compression. J Neurol Neurosurg Psychiatr 1987;50:151–4.
17. Heldmann U, Myschetzky PS, Thomsen HS. Frequency of unexpected multifocal metastasis in patients with acute spinal cord compression. Evaluation by low-field MR imaging in cancer patients. Acta Radiol 1997;38:372–5.
18. Helweg-Larsen S, Sorensen PS. Symptoms and signs in metastatic spinal cord compression: a study of progression from first symptom until diagnosis in 153 patients. Eur J Cancer 1994;30A:396–8.
19. Martenson JA Jr, Evans RG, Lie MR, et al. Treatment outcome and complications in patients treated for malignant epidural spinal cord compression (SCC). J Neurooncol 1985;3:77–84.
20. Torma T. Malignant tumors of the spine and spinal epidural space: a study based on 250 histologically verified cases. Acta Chir Scand Suppl 1957;225:1–176.
21. Loughrey GJ, Collins CD, Todd SM, et al. Magnetic resonance imaging in the management of suspected spinal canal disease in patients with known malignancy. Clin Radiol 2000;55:849–55.

22. Kienstra GE, Terwee CB, Dekker FW, et al. Prediction of spinal epidural metastases. Arch Neurol 2000;57:690–5.
23. Ruckdeschel JC. Early detection and treatment of spinal cord compression. Oncology (Williston Park) 2005;19:81–6 [discussion: 86].
24. Sorensen S, Helweg-Larsen S, Mouridsen H, et al. Effect of high-dose dexamethasone in carcinomatous metastatic spinal cord compression treated with radiotherapy: a randomised trial. Eur J Cancer 1994;30A:22–7.
25. Vecht CJ, Haaxma-Reiche H, van Putten WL, et al. Initial bolus of conventional versus high-dose dexamethasone in metastatic spinal cord compression. Neurology 1989;39:1255–7.
26. Barron KD, Hirano A, Araki S, et al. Experiences with metastatic neoplasms involving the spinal cord. Neurology 1959;9:91–106.
27. Constans JP, de Divitiis E, Donzelli R, et al. Spinal metastases with neurological manifestations. Review of 600 cases. J Neurosurg 1983;59:111–8.
28. Klimo P Jr, Thompson CJ, Kestle JR, et al. A meta-analysis of surgery versus conventional radiotherapy for the treatment of metastatic spinal epidural disease. Neuro Oncol 2005;7:64–76.
29. Maranzano E, Bellavita R, Rossi R, et al. Short-course versus split-course radiotherapy in metastatic spinal cord compression: results of a phase III, randomized, multicenter trial [see comment]. J Clin Oncol 2005;23:3358–65.
30. Rades D, Stalpers LJ, Veninga T, et al. Evaluation of five radiation schedules and prognostic factors for metastatic spinal cord compression. J Clin Oncol 2005;23: 3366–75.
31. Sze WM, Shelley MD, Held I, et al. Palliation of metastatic bone pain: single fraction versus multifraction radiotherapy—a systematic review of randomised trials. [see comment]. Clin Oncol (R Coll Radiol) 2003;15:345–52.
32. Peters LJ. The ESTRO Regaud lecture. Inherent radiosensitivity of tumor and normal tissue cells as a predictor of human tumor response. Radiother Oncol 1990;17:177–90.
33. Greenberg HS, Kim JH, Posner JB. Epidural spinal cord compression from metastatic tumor: results with a new treatment protocol. Ann Neurol 1980;8: 361–6.
34. Fourney DR, Abi-Said D, Lang FF, et al. Use of pedicle screw fixation in the management of malignant spinal disease: experience in 100 consecutive procedures. J Neurosurg 2001;94:25–37.
35. Gokaslan ZL, York JE, Walsh GL, et al. Transthoracic vertebrectomy for metastatic spinal tumors. J Neurosurg 1998;89:599–609.
36. Harrington KD. Anterior cord decompression and spinal stabilization for patients with metastatic lesions of the spine. J Neurosurg 1984;61:107–17.
37. Hosono N, Yonenobu K, Fuji T, et al. Vertebral body replacement with a ceramic prosthesis for metastatic spinal tumors. Spine 1995;20:2454–62.
38. North RB, LaRocca VR, Schwartz J, et al. Surgical management of spinal metastases: analysis of prognostic factors during a 10-year experience. J Neurosurg Spine 2005;2:564–73.
39. Overby MC, Rothman AS. Anterolateral decompression for metastatic epidural spinal cord tumors. Results of a modified costotransversectomy approach. J Neurosurg 1985;62:344–8.
40. Siegal T, Siegal T, Robin G, et al. Anterior decompression of the spine for metastatic epidural cord compression: a promising avenue of therapy? Ann Neurol 1982;11:28–34.

41. Siegal T, Tiqva P, Siegal T. Vertebral body resection for epidural compression by malignant tumors. Results of forty-seven consecutive operative procedures. J Bone Joint Surg Am 1985;67;375–82.

42. Sundaresan N, Galicich JH, Bains MS, et al. Vertebral body resection in the treatment of cancer involving the spine. Cancer 1984;53:1393–6.

43. Wang JC, Boland P, Mitra N, et al. Single-stage posterolateral transpedicular approach for resection of epidural metastatic spine tumors involving the vertebral body with circumferential reconstruction: results in 140 patients. Invited submission from the Joint Section Meeting on Disorders of the Spine and Peripheral Nerves, March 2004. J Neurosurg Spine 2004;1:287–98.

44. Weigel B, Maghsudi M, Neumann C, et al. Surgical management of symptomatic spinal metastases. Postoperative outcome and quality of life. Spine 1999;24:2240–6.

45. Young RF, Post EM, King GA. Treatment of spinal epidural metastases. Randomized prospective comparison of laminectomy and radiotherapy. J Neurosurg 1980;53:741–8.

46. Patchell RA, Tibbs PA, Regine WF, et al. Direct decompressive surgical resection in the treatment of spinal cord compression caused by metastatic cancer: a randomised trial [see comment]. Lancet 2005;366:643–8.

47. Tokuhashi Y, Matsuzaki H, Toriyama S, et al. Scoring system for the preoperative evaluation of metastatic spine tumor prognosis [see comment]. Spine 1990;15:1110–3.

48. Tomita K, Kawahara N, Kobayashi T, et al. Surgical strategy for spinal metastases [see comment]. Spine 2001;26:298–306.

49. van der Linden YM, Dijkstra SP, Vonk EJ, et al. Prediction of survival in patients with metastases in the spinal column: results based on a randomized trial of radiotherapy. Cancer 2005;103:320–8.

50. Bartels RH, Feuth T, van der Maazen R, et al. Development of a model with which to predict the life expectancy of patients with spinal epidural metastasis. Cancer 2007;110:2042–9.

51. Tokuhashi Y, Matsuzaki H, Oda H, et al. A revised scoring system for preoperative evaluation of metastatic spine tumor prognosis. Spine 2005;30:2186–91.

52. Chaichana KL, Woodworth GF, Sciubba DM, et al. Predictors of ambulatory function after decompressive surgery for metastatic epidural spinal cord compression. Neurosurgery 2008;62:683–92 [discussion: 683–92].

53. Jackson RJ, Loh SC, Gokaslan ZL. Metastatic renal cell carcinoma of the spine: surgical treatment and results [erratum appears in J Neurosurg 2001 Apr;94 (2 Suppl):340]. J Neurosurg 2001;94:18–24.

54. Ogihara S, Seichi A, Hozumi T, et al. Prognostic factors for patients with spinal metastases from lung cancer [see comment]. Spine 2006;31:1585–90.

55. Sciubba DM, Gokaslan ZL. Diagnosis and management of metastatic spine disease. Surg Oncol 2006;15:141–51.

56. Degen JW, Gagnon GJ, Voyadzis JM, et al. CyberKnife stereotactic radiosurgical treatment of spinal tumors for pain control and quality of life. J Neurosurg Spine 2005;2:540–9.

57. Fourney DR, Schomer DF, Nader R, et al. Percutaneous vertebroplasty and kyphoplasty for painful vertebral body fractures in cancer patients. J Neurosurg 2003;98:21–30.

58. Boogerd W, van der Sande JJ, Kroger R, et al. Effective systemic therapy for spinal epidural metastases from breast carcinoma. Eur J Cancer Clin Oncol 1989;25:149–53.

59. Sinoff CL, Blumsohn A. Spinal cord compression in myelomatosis: response to chemotherapy alone. Eur J Cancer Clin Oncol 1989;25:197–200.

Cerebral Edema, Altered Mental Status, Seizures, Acute Stroke, Leptomeningeal Metastases, and Paraneoplastic Syndrome

Denise M. Damek, MD[a,b,c],*

KEYWORDS

- Cerebral edema • Altered mental status
- Seizures • Acute stroke • Leptomeningeal metastases
- Paraneoplastic syndrome

Neurologic disorders are a frequent cause of emergency department (ED) visits, subspecialty consultation, and hospital admissions in oncology patients.[1–3] Neurologic disorders are often the presenting symptom of systemic cancer. In addition, neurologic complications are a source of significant disability, morbidity, and mortality in cancer patients. This article provides an overview of selected cancer-related neurologic emergencies that present to the ED, including cerebral edema and increased intracranial pressure, altered mental status, seizures, acute stroke, leptomeningeal metastases, and paraneoplastic neurologic syndromes.

CEREBRAL EDEMA AND INCREASED INTRACRANIAL PRESSURE

As a brain tumor enlarges, it produces focal findings by invasion and compression of surrounding brain tissue. More generalized signs and symptoms, such as headache,

---

[a] Neuro-Oncology, University of Colorado Denver School of Medicine, 12631 E. 17th Avenue, MS# B-185, Aurora, CO 80045, USA

[b] Department of Neurology, University of Colorado Denver School of Medicine, 12631 E. 17th Avenue, MS# B-185, Aurora, CO 80045, USA

[c] Department of Neurosurgery, University of Colorado Denver School of Medicine, 12631 E. 17th Avenue, MS# B-185, Aurora, CO 80045, USA

* Neuro-Oncology, University of Colorado Denver School of Medicine, 12631 E. 17th Avenue, MS# B-185, Aurora, CO 80045.

E-mail address: denise.damek@ucdenver.edu

Emerg Med Clin N Am 27 (2009) 209–229
doi:10.1016/j.emc.2009.02.003
0733-8627/09/$ – see front matter. Published by Elsevier Inc.

emed.theclinics.com

nausea, vomiting, papilledema, and depressed levels of consciousness, result from increased intracranial pressure due to the space occupied by the tumor mass, associated cerebral edema, or obstruction of cerebrospinal fluid outflow pathways.

Vasogenic edema occurs as tumor growth leads to disruption of the blood-brain barrier and increased capillary permeability, which allows a protein- and sodium-rich plasma filtrate to enter the extracellular fluid space and spread throughout adjacent white matter. Increased hydrostatic pressure within the tumor, an osmotic gradient, and the absence of a lymphatic system within the central nervous system also lead to extracellular fluid accumulation. As a result, focal mass effect, increased intracranial pressure, compromise of local blood supply, or brain herniation syndromes may occur.

Headaches are reported at presentation by approximately one half of all brain tumor patients, especially those with rapidly growing neoplasms or infratentorial tumors. At first glance these headaches may seem nondescript, but there are characteristics of headache in this patient population that the ED triage team will find valuable. Brain tumor patients generally describe a dull nonthrobbing headache similar to a tension headache. The headache is mild at onset, becoming increasingly more severe over days and weeks, and is typically associated with other symptoms of increased intracranial pressure and focal neurologic deficits. In fact, less than 10% of brain tumor patients have isolated headache syndromes, making the presence of abnormal neurologic signs and symptoms an important diagnostic distinction between tumor-related and benign headaches.[4] The classic brain tumor headache syndrome, characterized as a dull, aching pain that awakens the patient from sleep or is present on awakening with improvement thereafter, and often aggravated by positional change or Valsalva maneuvers, or associated with nausea and vomiting, is actually rare to nonexistent. Obstructive hydrocephalus is often associated with a more acute headache presentation and vomiting.

Patients with brain tumors may also experience headaches in conjunction with plateau pressure waves. Under normal circumstances, vasomotor tone automatically adjusts to maintain constant intracranial pressure with positional changes or other variables. However, in patients with brain tumors, mass effect and other factors can impede vasomotor autoregulation leading to plateau pressure waves that are characterized by the abrupt rapid elevation of intracranial pressure for brief 5- to 20-minute periods.[5] This sudden change in intracranial pressure produces short duration (20–30 minutes) headaches that are precipitated by a change in posture, and are often accompanied by an abrupt decline in mental status and emesis. Level of alertness is generally unaffected, but loss of consciousness can occur. These symptoms may be confused with seizure activity in patients with a known diagnosis of brain tumor.

Altered mental status is the initial symptom or sign in one third of brain tumor patients. Disturbances range from psychomotor retardation to lethargy to obtundation and coma. Papilledema is noted in approximately 8% of malignant glioma patients at presentation.[4] Most patients with papilledema do not report ocular symptoms, but some report transient visual obscurations or blurred vision. Visual acuity is generally unaffected. Early fundoscopic manifestations of papilledema include disc hyperemia, subtle edema of the nasal disc, small hemorrhages of the nerve fiber layer, and loss of spontaneous venous pulsations, which are normally present in 80% of the population. Later, the disc becomes grossly elevated, the margins obscure, and hemorrhage, exudates, and cotton wool spots may occur. Increased intracranial pressure may also cause vomiting, with or without nausea, as pressure is exerted on brain stem structures. Vague nonvertiginous dizziness is a frequent accompaniment. Projectile vomiting without nausea frequently occurs in patients with posterior fossa tumors and obstructive hydrocephalus.

Focal mass lesions can result in the asymmetric shift of brain contents from one intracranial compartment to another, producing herniation syndromes (**Table 1**). False localizing signs are more commonly seen with slow growing neoplasms that produce prolonged elevation of intracranial pressure and chronic tissue shift.[6] Acute herniation syndromes involving the medial temporal lobes (transtentorial herniation) or the cerebellar tonsils (tonsillar herniation), are often fatal and treatment outcomes, when successful, are poor. The earliest manifestation of transtentorial herniation is unilateral papillary dilatation and decrease in level of consciousness followed by ipsilateral or contralateral hemiparesis. Tonsillar herniation leads to compression of the respiratory centers in the medulla and ultimately respiratory arrest. Careful observation during recording of vital signs by the ED triage team may allow for the appreciation of warning signs of impending herniation such as abnormal breathing patterns (Cheyne-Stokes, central neurogenic hyperventilation, Biot's breathing), repetitive respiratory reflexes (sighing, yawning, hiccups), and Cushing's triad, which consists of bradycardia, hypertension, and change in respiratory pattern.

Currently there is no standard protocol or algorithm to guide the emergency medicine physician for the management of increased intracranial pressure or brain herniation. Likewise, there is a paucity of prospective clinical trial data on which to base management. General treatment approaches are contingent on rapidity and severity of neurologic symptoms, and vary widely from institution to institution. In some cases, medical management may reverse herniation syndromes, or serve to temporarily stabilize the patient until surgical decompression is possible.

Corticosteroids

Glucocorticoids, in particular dexamethasone, play a major role in the management of symptomatic cerebral edema.[7,8] Approximately 70% to 80% of brain tumor patients will experience symptom improvement following dexamethasone treatment.[9] In non-emergent clinical situations, the daily dose of dexamethasone ranges from 6 mg to 24 mg and is typically divided into 2 to 4 doses.[7] The long half-life of dexamethasone permits twice daily dosing, and the provision of 4 daily doses has become entrenched in current medical practice. In patients with impaired consciousness, rapidly progressing signs of increased intracranial pressure, or cerebral herniation, an intravenous bolus of dexamethasone (40–100 mg) followed by a maintenance dose of dexamethasone of 40 to 100 mg over 24 hours in divided doses may be effective in reversing symptoms. Concurrent provision of 20 mg of intravenous furosemide may further augment the effect of the steroid.

Physiologically, the first change after steroid administration is a decrease in plateau waves followed by a gradual decline in intracranial pressure over 48 to 72 hours.[10] Symptomatic improvement can be seen within the first few hours of intravenous steroid therapy, and maximal clinical improvement is generally achieved within 24 to 72 hours. Evidence of generalized brain dysfunction typically improves before focal neurologic symptoms or signs. If the desired clinical response is not achieved within 48 hours of standard dexamethasone dosing, the dose can be doubled every 48 hours until clinical response or a total daily dose of 100 mg of dexamethasone is reached.[11,12] The patient should then be maintained on the lowest dose necessary to maintain symptom control.

Hyperventilation

Intubation and hyperventilation to a target partial pressure of carbon dioxide (pCO_2) of 30 mm Hg remains the most rapid means of decreasing increased intracranial pressure. As the pCO_2 decreases, cerebral vasoconstriction in undamaged areas of the

Table 1
Brain herniation syndromes

Type of Herniation	Definition	Symptoms/Signs
Transtentorial herniation		
• Descending	Downward displacement of the brain through the tentorium at the level of the incisura	• Compression of ipsilateral cranial nerve III may lead to dilatation of the pupil and extraocular eye movement abnormalities • Compression of ipsilateral corticospinal tracts cause contralateral hemiparesis • Compression of the posterior cerebral artery may cause unilateral or bilateral occipital lobe infarction • Compression of the pontine perforating vessels may cause brain stem hemorrhage • Compression of the midbrain may cause hydrocephalus • Kernohan notch phenomenon is caused by compression of the contralateral cerebral peduncle against the adjacent tentorium causing false, localizing ipsilateral hemiparesis
• Ascending	Upward displacement of brain through the tentorium at the level of the incisura	• Depending on rapidity of shift, brain stem compression may cause nausea or vomiting, hydrocephalus, or rapid progression to coma
Subfalcine/cingulated herniation	Displacement of brain underneath the falx	• May be asymptomatic • Headache • Contralateral leg weakness • Compression of the anterior cerebral artery may cause ipsilateral frontal lobe infarction
Tonsillar herniation	Downward displacement of infratentorial brain through the foramen magnum	• Acute compression of the brain stem may cause obtundation, rapidly progressing to death • Insidious processes may cause Lhermitte phenomenon
Sphenoid/alar herniation	Supratentorial brain displaced anteriorly or posteriorly over the wing of the sphenoid bone	Frequently asymptomatic
• Anterior	Temporal lobe displaced anteriorly and superiorly over the sphenoid bone	—
• Posterior	Frontal lobe is displaced posteriorly and inferiorly over the sphenoid bone	—
Extracranial herniation	Displacement of brain through a cranial defect	Herniated brain may become ischemic

brain occurs, resulting in decreased cerebral blood volume and intracranial pressure. The benefit of hyperventilation manifests within 30 seconds and is maintained for about 15 to 20 minutes.[13] Thereafter, a compensatory metabolic acidosis negates its effect. The primary usefulness of hyperventilation is to gain immediate control of intracranial pressure, allowing time for other treatment modalities to take effect.

Osmotherapy

Hyperosmolar agents create an osmotic gradient that effectively draws water from the extracellular space to the higher osmolarity in blood, thereby reducing brain volume and intracranial pressure. Historically, mannitol is the most commonly used osmotic agent; however, there is growing evidence in support of the use of hypertonic saline.[14,15] Mannitol is typically provided as a 20% to 25% solution and given as a 0.5- to 2.0-g/kg intravenous loading dose. The effect of mannitol manifests within 15 to 30 minutes and is generally sustained for several hours.[13,16] If clinically warranted repeated small intravenous boluses may be administered, however, repeated doses of mannitol may precipitate rebound intracranial hypertension. The provision of a loop diuretic such as furosemide given 15 to 20 minutes after mannitol as a one time 20-mg intravenous dose may augment the benefit of mannitol.[17] Hypertonic saline at concentrations ranging from 3% to 23.4% seems to be as effective if not superior to mannitol with a more favorable side effect profile.[15,18–20] However, unlike mannitol, hypertonic saline is a significant vesicant, which should be preferentially infused into a central line.

Adjunct Therapies

Additional adjuncts to the management of increased intracranial pressure and acute herniation syndromes include elevation of the head, propofol or pentobarbital anesthesia, and hypothermia. Elevation of the head by 30 degrees with care to avoid flexion or extension of the neck maximizes venous outflow. Propofol induces vasoconstriction and decreases the cerebral metabolic rate of oxygen, which in turn reduces cerebral blood flow, cerebral blood volume, and intracranial pressure.[21] Barbiturates also suppress cerebral metabolism, which subsequently decreases cerebral blood flow and cerebral blood volumes. Hypothermia can reduce the cerebral metabolism rate of oxygen by 5% per degree reduction in core body temperature, thereby decreasing cerebral blood flow and intracranial pressure. However, increased risk of cardiac dysrhythmias, coagulopathy, and systemic infection limit its usefulness.

ALTERED MENTAL STATUS
Delirium

Delirium occurs in 25% to 40% of patients with cancer, and is present in up to 90% of terminally ill cancer patients.[22] Delirium, often used synonymously with acute confusion, is the most common cause of neurologic consultation in cancer patients, and results in upwards of 10% of admissions to general oncology wards.[2,22–24] The syndrome is characterized by rapid onset over hours or days of fluctuating abnormalities of thought, perception, and levels of awareness. More specifically, decreased attention and disorganized thinking are accompanied by variable altered level of consciousness, disorientation, decreased short term memory, hallucinations or illusions, alteration of sleep-wake cycle, and abnormal behavior modulation. Mood and behavior changes are often the primary outward manifestation of delirium. Patients may exhibit loud, boisterous, aggressive, and agitated behavior, or alternatively may have quiet, reserved, and passive behavior, and appear depressed. Brief simplistic psychotic ideas are commonly present, and neurologic signs such as unsteady gait and tremor may be seen.

Delirium often goes unrecognized, or may be confused with dementia, depression, psychoses, seizures, or attributed erroneously to terminal illness. In addition, it is consistently associated with more numerous and longer hospital stays, and increased morbidity and mortality.[24]

Delirium remains a clinical diagnosis. Although various instruments or assessment tools have been developed to screen patients for delirium, they remain largely unvalidated, unstudied, and unused in patients with cancer.[25] Key to recognition of delirium is a clear understanding of the patient's baseline cognitive functioning, as well as critical assessment of ongoing symptoms, which may require ancillary history from family members or other caregivers. In addition, a high index of suspicion, and awareness of associated risk factors and etiologies of delirium in the cancer patient is required of the ED team.

Delirium may result from direct and indirect effects of cancer and its treatment on the central nervous system. Multiple precipitating factors were identified in more than 60% of cancer patients with delirium, with a median number of 3 probable causes per patient.[22–24] The most common causes of delirium in the cancer patient included drugs, systemic infection, structural brain lesions, and metabolic dysfunction.[23,24] Metabolic aberrations included hyponatremia, hypoxia or hypoperfusion, and renal failure.[24] Cancer type and chemotherapy were not generally contributing factors.[24] In one report, low albumin levels were found in 80% of patients, but cachexia was not recorded and the extent of malnutrition was not known.[24] Similar to reports in noncancer patients, surgical procedures precipitated delirium in up to 40% of patients.[24,26] Likewise, infection was a strong risk factor for delirium, but it rarely occurred in isolation.[23,24] Data from elderly, noncancer patients found that delirium, not an elevated temperature, was frequently the first sign of sepsis.[27,28] Nonconvulsive status epilepticus (NCSE) may be an under-recognized cause of delirium in comatose patients.[29,30]

It is critical that the emergency medicine physician appreciates that delirium is reversible with appropriate intervention in more than 50% of patients.[22,24] Moreover, meaningful functional improvement can be seen in patients with advanced cancer if any reversible contributing factors are treated. Reversible precipitants of delirium include opioid and nonopioid psychoactive medications, dehydration, infection, surgical procedures, structural brain abnormalities, and NCSE.[22–24,29,31–33] Rapid improvement is frequently seen in patients with brain tumors or hemorrhagic metastases after administration of corticosteroids, which is often initiated in the ED.[24]

With few exceptions, the diagnostic evaluation of delirium in cancer patients does not differ from that routinely undertaken in noncancer patients. Neuroimaging is indicated in most cancer patients with delirium including those with a nonfocal examination, the exception being patients who rapidly clear following a medical intervention. Notably, lateralizing signs are absent in one fourth of patients with delirium and a structural brain lesion on neuroimaging.[24] Electroencephalography is indicated in comatose or significantly clouded patients; the reported incidence of NCSE in these patients is 6% to 8%.[29,30] In addition, because 3 or more contributory factors are often present, the diagnostic workup should not be truncated after the identification of one reasonable cause of delirium.

Overall, delirium is a poor prognostic factor in cancer patients. Statistically significant decreases in median survival are reported in cancer patients with delirium compared with those without delirium, especially if the acute confusion is attributable to structural brain lesions or multiple toxic or metabolic abnormalities.[22,34–36]

Nonconvulsive Status Epilepticus

NCSE has been reported to be the underlying cause of altered mental status in up to 6% of cancer patients.[29,30] A high index of suspicion is required for the diagnosis of NCSE, in part due to its variable and nonspecific presentation, its lack of associated motor activity, and the absence of a prior history of epilepsy or seizures in most patients at presentation. NCSE is classically defined as a state of continuous or intermittent seizure activity without return to baseline lasting at least 30 minutes. More recently, the Epilepsy Research Foundation defined NCSE as a range of conditions in which electrographic seizure activity is prolonged, resulting in nonconvulsive clinical symptoms.[37]

The one consistent clinical symptom of NCSE is fluctuating altered mental status; however, even then, symptoms can encompass a spectrum ranging from psychomotor retardation to mild confusion to depressed consciousness. Motor manifestations are often limited to focal myoclonic jerks involving the face, eyelids, or extremities, however brief tonic or clonic movements of one or multiple extremities may also occur. Additional possible manifestations include head deviation, automatisms, and eye movement abnormalities including hippus, nystagmoid eye movements, repeated blinking, and persistent eye deviation. In one prospective study, the combination of a remote risk factor for seizures (previous stroke, neurosurgical procedure, brain tumor, or history of meningitis) and ocular movement abnormalities on neurologic examination had 100% sensitivity for NCSE, but low specificity.[38]

In some cases, imaging findings may support the diagnosis of NCSE. Characteristic cortical ribbon hyperintensity on long repetition time (TR)-weighted magnetic resonance sequences or diffusion weighted imaging sequences, with or without leptomeningeal enhancement was reported in 4 of 8 patients with NCSE in one series.[39] Imaging findings did not respect vascular territories, lacked mass effect, and either resolved or improved on follow-up imaging studies.[39]

Emergent electroencephalography (EEG) is recommended for patients with suspected NCSE. If an emergent EEG is not possible, an empirical trial of intravenous lorazepam should be considered given the tolerable risk of lorazepam compared with the benefit of potential prevention of secondary cerebral damage.

SEIZURES

New onset seizures herald the diagnosis of central nervous system brain tumors in 20% to 40% of patients, and account for 10% to 15% of adult-onset seizures.[40,41] Furthermore, seizures occur at some point in the clinical course in 40% to 60% of patients with gliomas, in 30% to 40% of patients with brain metastases, and in approximately 13% of all cancer patients.[3,40,42] Seizure risk varies depending on the tumor type and location, patient age, and tumor treatment.[42] Slow-growing tumors that involve or abut the cerebral cortex are associated with a higher incidence of seizures.[43]

In many cases, a clinical diagnosis of seizure is established after the patient history and examination is performed. However, disorders such as syncope, migraine, medication effects, and nonepileptic spells, may be confused with seizures. In addition, the diagnosis of NCSE is often overlooked in the ED. Head computed tomography (CT) and routine EEG should be considered as part of the neurodiagnostic evaluation of adult patients with unprovoked first seizure in the emergency department.[44,45] Brain imaging results in an acute management change in approximately 10% to 15% of these patients and EEG demonstrates significant abnormalities in approximately one third of patients, and provides risk assessment for seizure recurrence.[44,45]

Seizures associated with brain tumors and other structural lesions are most often simple partial or complex partial seizures. Secondarily generalized seizures may occur, but the focal onset of these seizures often goes unnoticed by the patient or witnesses. Postictal deficits (Todd's paralysis) are more common in patients with structural brain lesions and may be prolonged.[46] Whereas convulsive status epilepticus is rare in patients with brain tumors, it is fatal in 6% to 35%.[47] In contrast to structural seizures in brain tumor patients, seizures related to metabolic abnormalities are typically generalized seizures. Standard of care diagnostic evaluation and seizure management is appropriate in the brain tumor patient with the following specific considerations.

Many physicians endorse the prophylactic use of anticonvulsant medications in brain tumor patients who have never had a seizure, citing the high frequency of seizures in this patient population and the low risk of seizure medications. However, the emergency medicine physician must appreciate the lack of evidence that prophylactic anticonvulsant medications will prevent seizures in these patients, and that seizure medications are not without potential side effects and drug interactions. Phenytoin, a commonly prescribed anticonvulsant medication, causes a morbilliform rash in approximately 20% of brain tumor patients. Stevens-Johnson syndrome is rare, but is seen more often with the combination of radiation therapy, steroid taper, and phenytoin.[48] Even minor side effects of antiepileptic drug can negatively impact quality of life of patients already undergoing aggressive antitumor therapy. In addition, enzyme-inducing anticonvulsant medications may interact with chemotherapy and other drugs. For this reason, the use of nonenzyme-inducing anticonvulsant medications is preferable. Practice parameters issued by the American Academy of Neurology (AAN) currently recommend withholding prophylactic anticonvulsants in brain tumor patients who have never had a seizure.[42]

A related issue is the provision of prophylactic anticonvulsant medications in the setting of neurosurgical procedures. Traditionally, neurosurgeons prescribe prophylactic anticonvulsant medications before and for 6 to 12 weeks after neurosurgical procedures. The AAN practice guidelines recommend the tapering and discontinuance of anticonvulsant medications after the first postoperative week in brain tumor patients without known seizures.[42]

The etiology of provoked seizures in cancer patients is similar to that of the general population. However, some causes are particularly linked to cancer therapies. One such example is reversible posterior leukoencephalopathy syndrome (RPLS), also known as posterior reversible encephalopathy syndrome. RPLS in cancer patients is associated with numerous chemotherapeutic agents, especially cisplatin. RPLS has also been reported following the administration of 5-fluorouracil, bleomycin, vinblastine, vincristine, etoposide, paclitaxel, ifosfamide, cyclophosphamide, doxorubicin, cytarabine, methotrexate, oxaliplatin, and bevacizumab.[49–51]

The classic presentation of RPLS is the development of a subacute syndrome of headache, altered consciousness, generalized seizures, and visual disturbances, occurring in conjunction with posterior cerebral white matter vasogenic edema on CT/MRI.[52] Typically the syndrome manifests over several days, but a more acute presentation may occur. Altered consciousness may vary from excessive drowsiness to coma, seizures may be focal or generalized, and visual disturbances range from blurred vision to cortical blindness. Additional neurologic symptoms such as paresis may also be present. Moderate to severe hypertension occurs in approximately 75% of patients. Hypertension typically develops at the same time as neurologic symptoms, but occasionally it may precede the clinical manifestations of RPLS.[53,54]

Radiographically, MRI typically demonstrates symmetric hemispheric edema in the parietal and occipital lobes involving cortical and subcortical white matter, approximating the border zone vascular territory.[54] Although involvement of the parietal and occipital lobes occurs most often, similar radiographic abnormalities can be located in the frontal lobes, the inferior temporal-occipital junction, and the cerebellum. Focal areas of restricted diffusion are seen in less than one fourth of patients. Approximately 15% of patients have radiographic evidence of hemorrhage in the form of focal hematoma, or isolated sulcal or subarachnoid blood.[54]

ACUTE STROKE

Ischemic, hemorrhagic, and thrombotic cerebrovascular disease occurs in approximately 15% of cancer patients, but only one half of cancer patients experience symptoms referable to their lesions.[55] Most cerebrovascular disease associated with hematologic cancer is hemorrhagic, whereas in solid tumors there is an even division between infarction and hemorrhage.[55]

Cerebral infarction occurs infrequently in hematologic malignancies, and is generally hemorrhagic. Leukemic patients may develop septic emboli, infarction related to disseminated intravascular coagulation, or venous infarctions related to cerebral venous thrombosis. Most cerebral infarction in patients with lymphoma is attributable to disseminated intravascular coagulation or nonbacterial thrombotic endocarditis (NBTE).

Most strokes in patients with solid tumors are embolic and tend to occur late in the patient's clinical course. Rarely, stroke can be the presenting symptom of occult malignancy.[56–58] NBTE is frequently cited as the most common cause of stroke in cancer patients, and some propose that cancer-specific factors such as tumor type and associated coagulation disorders are more determinant of stroke risk in cancer patients than the classic atherosclerotic stroke risk factors.[55,59] However, supporting data are inconsistent. Whereas some reports attribute a disproportionately small number of strokes in cancer patients, less than 20%, to atherosclerotic disease, other studies report no significant difference in atherosclerotic stroke incidence between cancer stroke patients and noncancer stroke patients.[55,59–62] Overall, the ED physician must consider typical ischemic stroke mechanisms as well as disease-specific stroke risk factors in the cancer patient. The more common cancer-related stroke mechanisms are discussed in the following subsections.

Nonbacterial Thrombotic Endocarditis

NBTE is characterized by the presence of cardiac valve vegetation formed by fibrin and platelet aggregates, occurring in the absence of infection or inflammation. Involvement of left-sided heart valves (aortic more often than mitral) is more common than right-sided heart valves.[63] The vegetation is typically small, irregular, and easily friable with a strong propensity to embolize.[64] Not surprisingly, the most common presenting symptom, occurring in approximately 50% of patients, is recurrent systemic emboli to cerebral, coronary, renal, and mesenteric bed circulations or the extremities, respectively producing acute stroke, myocardial infarction, hematuria, abdominal pain, or cold, cyanotic, or pulseless limbs.[63,64] Symptomatic valvular dysfunction is uncommon.

NBTE is most commonly associated with widely disseminated mucin-producing adenocarcinomas of the lung or gastrointestinal tract and lymphoma.[64,65] Approximately 70% of patients have coexistent disseminated intravascular coagulation.[66] Autopsy data suggest that NBTE often goes undiagnosed in the clinical setting, reflecting the difficulty in establishing a definitive diagnosis.[59] The diagnostic gold standard is the demonstration of valvular vegetation on transesophageal echocardiogram in the absence of positive blood cultures. However, due to the nature of the vegetation and its propensity to embolize, transesophageal echocardiogram may not detect the remaining small, fragmented vegetation. Additional clues may be of diagnostic importance in the cancer patient. Whereas cardiac murmurs are uncommon in NBTE, their presence in a cancer patient should raise a diagnostic suspicion of NBTE. Likewise, abnormal coagulation studies, including prothrombin time, partial thromboplastin time, fibrinogen, thrombin time, D-dimer, and cross-linked fibrin degradation products are suggestive of NBTE in the appropriate clinical setting. The distribution of strokes on brain MRI may be helpful in differentiating NBTE from septic emboli. One small study found that strokes due to NBTE involved multiple, widespread, small and large arteries, as opposed to a single lesion, multiple lesions within a single arterial territory, or multiple punctate disseminated lesions—all patterns more suggestive of septic emboli.[67] If feasible, the treatment of NBTE is typically life-long anticoagulation with intravenous or subcutaneous heparin.[68] Warfarin often fails to control the coagulopathy and is associated with recurrent thromboembolic events.[68] There are insufficient data for comment on the efficacy of the newer antico-agulant agents such as fondaparinux.

Therapy-Induced Stroke

Cerebrovascular disease may be provoked by cancer therapy. In fact, cancer treatment accounts for most strokes in patients with a primary brain tumor. Approximately 20% to 60% of strokes in this patient population are the result of intraoperative vascular injury and occur adjacent to the resection bed.[62,69] In addition, brain irradiation commonly causes accelerated atherosclerosis and small vessel arteriopathy within the radiated field, which may cause stroke or transient ischemic attacks in medium to large vessels typically occurring 6 months to 5 years following radiation treatment.[62,70,71] Conventional atherosclerotic stroke management is appropriate in these patients.

Ischemic stroke occurs in less than 1% of cancer patients receiving chemotherapy, primarily L-asparaginase, cisplatin, 5-fluorouracil, and methotrexate.[72–75] Mechanisms include thrombosis, vasospasm, thrombocytopenia, and decreased renewal capacity of endothelial cells. Despite the wide range of proposed causes, the vascular events related to chemotherapy almost always occur within days to 1 month of therapy.

Tumor Emboli

Solid tumors rarely produce stroke as the result of tumor emboli to cerebral arteries, compression or invasion of a cerebral artery, or compression of cerebral sinuses causing venous infarction.[76,77] The most common sources of tumor emboli are atrial myxomas and other cardiac tumors, as well as lung cancer. Lung tumor emboli most often occur within 48 hours of surgical manipulation of lung tissue, but may also result from tumor invasion of the pulmonary veins or left atrium of the heart.[76] Signs and symptoms of emboli to multiple body organs or the extremities are frequently seen. Stroke from lung tumor emboli should be suspected in any patient with primary or metastatic lung cancer who develops stroke in the immediate postoperative period or has evidence of multi-organ infarction. Treatment must address tumor growth at the embolic infarction site and the primary tumor.

Septic Emboli

Leukemia patients are particularly susceptible to septic infarction from fungal or bacterial sepsis and infectious vasculitis. Agranulocytosis during and after therapy predisposes these patients to fungal infection, in particular *Aspergillus* or *Candida* sp.[78] *Aspergillus* pulmonary infection facilitates hematogenous dissemination of these microorganisms, and their large hyphae may become trapped with the lumen of medium- to large-sized vessels, causing cerebral infarction and focal neurologic deficits.[79] Infarctions are often multiple, may be hemorrhagic, and may evolve into cerebral abscess. Chest roentgenograms or CT scans often indicate infection, and patients may be febrile. Blood and sputum cultures are typically negative. Transbronchial biopsy or brain biopsy is often necessary to establish the diagnosis. Antifungal therapy is often ineffective and patients generally succumb to progressive infection.

Hemorrhagic Cerebral Metastases

Hemorrhage into cerebral metastases in patients with melanoma, germ cell, and non-small-cell lung carcinoma primaries account for most hemorrhagic cerebrovascular disease in patients with solid tumors.[55] Thrombocytopenia-related intracranial hemorrhage occurs less commonly. Hemorrhage into a solid tumor causes acute strokelike symptoms in two thirds of patients and subacute focal neurologic symptoms suggestive of an enlarging mass lesion in one third of patients. In contrast to primary intracerebral hemorrhage, corticosteroids are beneficial in intratumoral hemorrhage.[80] Surgical evacuation of the clot may be indicated to reduce increased intracranial pressure. Additional treatment addresses the underlying metastatic disease.

Pituitary Apoplexy

Pituitary apoplexy is an acute, potentially life-threatening clinical syndrome caused by the acute expansion of a hypophyseal adenoma as a result of hemorrhage or infarction. It occurs in 0.6% to 17% of patients with pituitary adenoma, in particular chromophobic and eosinophilic adenomas.[81,82] However, intralesional hemorrhage or infarct may be asymptomatic and only evident on radiographic studies or at microscopic examination. Apoplexy is rarely the presenting symptom of a pituitary adenoma.[81,83] Predisposing factors include conditions that either reduce or acutely increase blood flow in the pituitary gland, hormonal stimulation of the pituitary gland, or anticoagulated states.[84]

Clinically, acute expansion of the pituitary gland and compression of perisellar structures may cause severe headaches, nausea, vomiting, visual disturbances, ophthalmoplegia, and decreased level of consciousness. Long-standing pituitary gland compression may result in hypopituitarism. Prompt surgical decompression is indicated in acutely symptomatic cases.[83] Medical management may be considered in appropriate tumor subtypes with more indolent clinical presentations.

LEPTOMENINGEAL METASTASES

Leptomeningeal metastases (LM) occurs in up to 8% of all cancer patients, and in 5% to 20% of cancer patients with widely metastatic disease.[85,86] Primary brain tumors, such as primary lymphomas, medulloblastomas, and germ cell tumors of the central nervous system, may have LM at initial diagnosis.[87] Otherwise, LM rarely occurs in patients without evidence of widespread systemic disease.[88,89] Any systemic cancer can spread to the leptomeninges; however, LM is most commonly associated with leukemia, non-Hodgkin lymphoma, breast carcinoma, non-small-cell lung cancer, and melanoma.[90–92]

The clinical hallmark of LM is the presence of symptoms and signs referable to multiple sites within the central nervous system, cranial nerves, and spinal roots. Not surprisingly, the presentation of LM is highly variable and diagnosis requires a high index of suspicion. Virtually any nervous system abnormality may occur; however, some symptoms are seen more consistently. Approximately 60% of patients with LM report weakness and paresthesia of the lower extremities indicating lumbosacral nerve root involvement, and more than 70% will have corresponding spinal signs of asymmetric weakness, sensory loss, and depressed reflexes. One half of patients manifest nonspecific cerebral symptoms including headache, nausea and vomiting, and cognitive changes. Meningismus and nuchal rigidity are present in only 15% of patients. One third of patients have cranial nerve dysfunction. In decreasing frequency, patients have symptoms and signs of oculomotor, facial, auditory, optic, trigeminal, and hypoglossal nerve dysfunction.[90–92] Papilledema may occur in the setting of communicating hydrocephalus. Uncommon manifestations of LM include diabetes insipidus, central hypoventilation, cerebral infarction, NCSE, and psychiatric symptoms.[93]

A definitive diagnosis of LM requires identification of malignant cells in the cerebrospinal fluid (CSF). Two or 3 samplings of CSF may be required before malignant cells are detected; the diagnostic yield of CSF samples obtained in the ED can be optimized through the collection of at least 10 mL of CSF for cytologic examination, and the prompt delivery of the specimen to the laboratory. Characteristic CSF abnormalities in LM include an elevated opening pressure in more than 50% of patients, mononuclear pleocytosis in more than 70% of patients, elevated protein in approximately 80% of patients, and decreased glucose in 25% to 30% of patients. The range of CSF protein elevation in LM is wide with a median total protein concentration of 1 g/L.[94]

In some cases, a presumptive diagnosis of LM is made on the basis of appropriate clinical symptoms and signs and neuroimaging findings consistent with LM in known cancer patients. MRI diagnosis of LM has up to 65% sensitivity and 77% specificity.[93] MR findings in LM may be normal or may demonstrate communicating hydrocephalus, effacement of the sulci and cisterns, linear or nodular subependymal, leptomeningeal, nerve root, or dural enhancement, and diffuse thickening of spinal nerve roots.[95] Diffuse leptomeningeal enhancement can also occur with cerebral hypotension following lumbar puncture, and may be misinterpreted as radiographic evidence of LM.[96] For this reason, if feasible, MRI should be obtained before lumbar puncture.

The overall prognosis of LM is poor; however, the cause of death in these patients is most often widespread uncontrolled systemic disease, not LM. As a consequence, the primary expectation of treatment is improved quality of life and prolonged time to neurologic progression.[97] The treatment of LM must address the entire neuroaxis and relies on a combination of radiation, chemotherapy, and supportive care. Radiation provides the most effective symptom relief and therapy for bulky tumor deposits. However, irradiation of the entire neuroaxis is generally too toxic in heavily pretreated patients. Chemotherapy provided by either intrathecal (IT) injection or systemic routes on occasion addresses LM disease throughout the entire neuroaxis.[97–99] However, impairment of CSF flow, which occurs in up to 70% of patients with LM, can impede uniform IT chemotherapy distribution and is a significant factor in drug failure.[100] Therefore, a combined approach is typically used consisting of chemotherapy and focal irradiation targeting regions of bulky disease, symptomatic levels of the neuroaxis, and regions of subarachnoid CSF block.[101]

Acute therapy complications frequently prompt ED evaluation. The most common complication, aseptic meningitis, clinically mimics bacterial meningitis. Similar to bacterial meningitis, CSF analysis shows pleocytosis and elevated protein. However, aseptic meningitis occurs within hours to 1 day following IT drug administration, much earlier than one would see iatrogenic bacterial meningitis. Symptoms generally resolve within a few days and treatment is symptomatic with antipyretics, antiemetics, and steroids. Aseptic meningitis may occur following the first IT drug dose or after any number of cycles. The syndrome often does not recur and further IT treatment may be provided.

Acute encephalopathy characterized by seizures, altered mental status, and lethargy, may occur within 24 to 48 hours of IT MTX or AraC. The treatment is symptomatic and symptoms generally resolve completely. In addition, concurrent IT chemotherapy and spinal irradiation may cause a transverse myelopathy. Back or leg pain, paraplegia, sensory loss, and bowel/bladder dysfunction typically develop within 48 hours of IT chemotherapy, but may occur within 30 minutes or up to 2 weeks following treatment. CSF is found to have elevated protein levels and MRI shows expansion of the spinal cord and hyperintensity on T2-weighted sequences. The prognosis for recovery is poor with persistent paraparesis in approximately 60% of those affected.

PARANEOPLASTIC NEUROLOGIC SYNDROMES

Paraneoplastic neurologic syndromes (PNS) are a collective group of disorders occurring in patients with cancer as a remote effect of the malignancy. These syndromes cannot be attributed directly to the tumor or its metastases, to cancer therapies, or to cancer-associated infection, vascular or coagulation disorders, nutritional deficits, or metabolic abnormalities (**Table 2**). PNS develop in 3% to 5% of patients with small-cell lung cancer, in 15% to 20% with thymomas, and in 3% to 10% with B cell or plasma cell neoplasms.[102] They occur in less than 1% of other tumor types.[102] Overall, PNS are diagnosed in less than 0.01% of cancer patients.[103] However, despite their rarity, paraneoplastic disorders have a significant impact on oncology patients not only because they antedate the diagnosis of cancer in up to 80% of affected individuals but also because they frequently cause significant disability due to early onset and irreversible destruction of neural tissues.[104] Prompt recognition of PNS by the emergency medicine physician will help facilitate an accurate diagnosis, allowing treatment of the underlying tumor at an early stage, and potentially mitigating neurologic disability.

Critical to the diagnosis of PNS is the recognition of a specific group of neurologic syndromes, referred to as classic PNS, that are highly suggestive, but not diagnostic, of a paraneoplastic origin. These classic PNS include Lambert-Eaton myasthenic syndrome, subacute cerebellar degeneration, limbic encephalitis, sensory neuronopathy, opsoclonus-myoclonus, dermatomyositis, stiff-person syndrome, retinopathy, encephalomyelitis, and chronic gastrointestinal pseudo-obstruction. However, it is important for the emergency medicine physician to recognize that most patients with these syndromes do not harbor an underlying malignancy. Approximately 50% of patients with Lambert-Eaton myasthenic syndrome or subacute cerebellar degeneration have an underlying tumor, whereas the incidence of malignancy in the remaining classic PNS is less than 20%.[104] Several factors implicate paraneoplastic origin. The presence of risk factors for malignancy such as smoking or family history, or symptoms associated with malignancy such as unexplained weight loss or night sweats, warrants consideration of a paraneoplastic origin. The presentation and disease course of PNS is often dramatic compared with the corresponding non–tumor-related syndromes. PNS typically have a subacute symptom onset with a rapidly progressive clinical course and early onset of severe disability.[105] In addition,

Table 2
Classic paraneoplastic neurologic syndromes

Classic PNS	Onset	Primary Clinical Symptoms and Signs
Limbic encephalitis	Subacute over weeks to months	o Short term memory loss that may progress to dementia o Personality changes o Anxiety, depression. agitation o Confusion o Olfactory and gustatory hallucinations o Partial or generalized seizures o Sleep disturbances
Subacute cerebellar degeneration	Subacute over weeks to months	o Initially patients note gait instability, then rapid evolution to truncal and limb ataxia o Dysarthria and dysphagia o Diplopia and nystagmus
Opsoclonus-myoclonus	Fairly acute over days to weeks	o Opsoclonus (almost continuous involuntary, arrhythmic, multidirectional chaotic rapid eye movements, that persist during eye closure and sleep) o Myoclonic jerks of limbs and trunk o Mild encephalopathy
Cancer-associated retinopathy (CAR)	Subacute over weeks to months	o Painless vision loss progressing to blindness over 6 to 18 months o Photopsias (flickering lights) o Peripheral and ring scotomatas
Melanoma-associated retinopathy(MAR)	Acute over days	o Shimmering or flickering light phenomena o Night blindness o Midperipheral visual field loss
Stiff-person syndrome	Insidious	o Rigidity of axial and proximal limb muscles with cocontraction of agonist and antagonist muscles o Intermittent painful spasms precipitated by sensory stimuli o Symptoms are absent during sleep and anesthesia

Subacute sensory neuronopathy	Subacute	○ Asymmetric pain and paresthesias involving the arms more than the legs ○ Pain is later replaced by numbness, limb ataxia, and pseudoathetotic movements of the hands ○ Facial numbness, sensorineural deafness, and sensory abnormalities of the trunk may also occur ○ Absent deep tendon reflexes and involvement of all sensory modalities especially joint position and vibratory senses
Chronic gastrointestinal pseudo-obstruction	Subacute	○ Severe constipation ○ Weight loss ○ Abdominal distension ○ Dysphagia ○ Nausea and vomiting
Lambert-Eaton myasthenic syndrome	Subacute	○ Proximal muscle weakness, legs more than arms. Symptoms are out of proportion to weakness. Strength may initially improve after exercise then decrease with sustained activity. ○ Deep tendon reflexes are reduced or absent, but may transiently improve after exercise. ○ Mild autonomic dysfunction ○ Mild ptosis/ophthalmoplegia
Dermatomyositis	Slowly progressive over months	○ Symmetric proximal muscle weakness ○ Associated cutaneous manifestations include a heliotrope rash involving the periorbital skin, erythematous scaly plaques on dorsal hands, periungual telangiectasia, Gottron's papules, and a photosensitive poikilodermatous eruption

syndromic overlap is frequently seen in PNS, but uncommon in disorders unrelated to cancer.

By definition, a paraneoplastic neurologic disorder requires the presence of an underlying malignancy, generally within 5 years of its diagnosis. Most patients do not have an established cancer diagnosis at presentation; however, the underlying cancer is discovered in 70% to 80% of patients at the initial cancer screening or within 4 to 6 months.[102] The risk of developing cancer significantly decreases after 2 years and becomes remote after 5 years. CT of the chest, abdomen, and pelvis or fluoro-deoxyglucose positron emission tomography are the most commonly used screening tests for malignancy in cases of suspected PNS.

In many cases, patients with PNS may either present with a nonclassic neurologic syndrome or have no identifiable tumor. In these scenarios, the identification of a well-characterized paraneoplastic antibody facilitates the definite diagnosis of PNS. Although numerous paraneoplastic or onconeural antibodies are currently under investigation for a purported relationship with PNS, only a few have been well charac-terized, including anti-Hu (antinuclear neuronal antibody type 1 or ANNA-1), anti-Yo (Purkinje cell antibody type 1 or PCA-1), anti-Ri (ANNA-2), anti-CV2/CRMP5, anti-Ma proteins, and anti-amphyphysin. However, up to 50% of patients with an established PNS diagnosis do not have detectable paraneoplastic antibodies.[105] Additional corrob-orating clinical evidence is required to establish a diagnosis of possible PNS in those patients with clinically suspected PNS that does not meet the diagnostic criteria.

Aside from onconeural antibodies, the diagnostic workup for paraneoplastic disor-ders yields fairly nonspecific findings of central nervous system inflammation, and, most importantly, serves to exclude alternative disorders. CSF evaluation may show mild pleocytosis, elevated protein, and oligoclonal bands. Histopathologic tissue examination demonstrates a nonspecific T cell infiltration.[102] Brain MRI is typically normal. However, hyperintensity on long TR sequences involving the mesial temporal lobes can be seen in limbic encephalitis. More widespread abnormalities, with addi-tional involvement of the brain stem, may be seen in patients with encephalomyelitis. Cerebellar atrophy is a late finding in subacute cerebellar degeneration.

To date, there are no evidence-based recommendations for treatment of PNS. Successful treatment of the underlying malignancy is by far the most effective treat-ment strategy for the stabilization of neurologic deficits from PNS. Immune therapy is often beneficial for PNS affecting the peripheral nervous system, neuromuscular junction, and muscle, and may consist of steroids, intravenous immunoglobulin, or plasma exchange. Central nervous system paraneoplastic disorders are more refrac-tory to treatment, although there are anecdotal reports of response to steroids or intra-venous immunoglobulin, as well as spontaneous remission. Symptomatic treatment of seizures, psychiatric manifestations, movement disorders, and so forth is indicated.

REFERENCES

1. Swenson KK, Rose MA, Ritz L, et al. Recognition and evaluation of oncology-related symptoms in the emergency department. Ann Emerg Med 1995;26:12–7.
2. Gilbert MR, Grossman SA. Incidence and nature of neurologic problems in patients with solid tumors. Am J Med 1986;81:951–4.
3. Clouston PD, DeAngelis LM, Posner JB. The spectrum of neurological disease in patients with systemic cancer. Ann Neurol 1992;31:268–73.
4. Black P, Wen P. Clinical, imaging and laboratory diagnosis of brain tumors. In: Kaye AH, Laws E Jr, editors. Brain tumors. New York: Churchill Livingstone; 1995. p. 191–214.

5. Matsuda M, Yoneda S, Handa H, et al. Cerebral hemodynamic changes during plateau waves in brain-tumor patients. J Neurosurg 1979;50:483–8.
6. Gassel MM. False localizing signs. A review of the concept and analysis of the occurrence in 250 cases of intracranial meningioma. Arch Neurol 1961;4: 526–54.
7. Sarin R, Murthy V. Medical decompressive therapy for primary and metastatic intracranial tumours. Lancet Neurol 2003;2:357–65.
8. Weissman DE. Glucocorticoid treatment for brain metastases and epidural spinal cord compression: a review. J Clin Oncol 1988;6:543–51.
9. Ruderman NB, Hall TC. Use of glucocorticoids in the palliative treatment of metastatic brain tumors. Cancer 1965;18:298–306.
10. Alberti E, Hartmann A, Schutz HJ, et al. The effect of large doses of dexamethasone on the cerebrospinal fluid pressure in patients with supratentorial tumors. J Neurol 1978;217:173–81.
11. Lieberman A, LeBrun Y, Glass P, et al. Use of high dose corticosteroids in patients with inoperable brain tumours. J Neurol Neurosurg Psychiatr 1977;40: 678–82.
12. Renaudin J, Fewer D, Wilson CB, et al. Dose dependency of decadron in patients with partially excised brain tumors. J Neurosurg 1973;39:302–5.
13. Ropper AH, Gress DR, Diringer MN, et al. Management of intracranial pressure and mass effect. In: Ropper AH, editor. Neurological and neurosurgical intensive care. 4th edition. Philadelphia: Lippincott Williams & Wilkins; 2003. p. 26–51.
14. The Brain Trauma Foundation. The American Association of Neurological Surgeons. The Joint Section on Neurotrauma and Critical Care. Use of mannitol. J Neurotrauma 2000;17:521–5.
15. Koenig MA, Bryan M, Lewin JL 3rd, et al. Reversal of transtentorial herniation with hypertonic saline. Neurology 2008;70:1023–9.
16. Ravussin P, Abou-Madi M, Archer D, et al. Changes in CSF pressure after mannitol in patients with and without elevated CSF pressure. J Neurosurg 1988;69:869–76.
17. Pollay M, Fullenwider C, Roberts PA, et al. Effect of mannitol and furosemide on blood-brain osmotic gradient and intracranial pressure. J Neurosurg 1983;59: 945–50.
18. Vialet R, Albanese J, Thomachot L, et al. Isovolume hypertonic solutes (sodium chloride or mannitol) in the treatment of refractory posttraumatic intracranial hypertension: 2 mL/kg 7.5% saline is more effective than 2 mL/kg 20% mannitol. Crit Care Med 2003;31:1683–7.
19. Qureshi AI, Suarez JI. Use of hypertonic saline solutions in treatment of cerebral edema and intracranial hypertension. Crit Care Med 2000;28:3301–13.
20. Suarez JI, Qureshi AI, Bhardwaj A, et al. Treatment of refractory intracranial hypertension with 23.4% saline. Crit Care Med 1998;26:1118–22.
21. Alkire MT, Haier RJ, Barker SJ, et al. Cerebral metabolism during propofol anesthesia in humans studied with positron emission tomography. Anesthesiology 1995;82:393–403 [discussion: 27A].
22. Lawlor PG, Gagnon B, Mancini IL, et al. Occurrence, causes, and outcome of delirium in patients with advanced cancer: a prospective study. Arch Intern Med 2000;160:786–94.
23. Doriath V, Paesmans M, Catteau G, et al. Acute confusion in patients with systemic cancer. J Neurooncol 2007;83:285–9.
24. Tuma R, DeAngelis LM. Altered mental status in patients with cancer. Arch Neurol 2000;57:1727–31.

25. Weinrich S, Sarna L. Delirium in the older person with cancer. Cancer 1994;74: 2079–91.
26. Marcantonio ER, Goldman L, Mangione CM, et al. A clinical prediction rule for delirium after elective noncardiac surgery. JAMA 1994;271:134–9.
27. Francis J, Martin D, Kapoor WN. A prospective study of delirium in hospitalized elderly. JAMA 1990;263:1097–101.
28. Schor JD, Levkoff SE, Lipsitz LA, et al. Risk factors for delirium in hospitalized elderly. JAMA 1992;267:827–31.
29. Cocito L, Audenino D, Primavera A. Altered mental state and nonconvulsive status epilepticus in patients with cancer. Arch Neurol 2001;58:1310.
30. Towne AR, Waterhouse EJ, Boggs JG, et al. Prevalence of nonconvulsive status epilepticus in comatose patients. Neurology 2000;54:340–5.
31. Maddocks I, Somogyi A, Abbott F, et al. Attenuation of morphine-induced delirium in palliative care by substitution with infusion of oxycodone. J Pain Symptom Manage 1996;12:182–9.
32. de Stoutz ND, Bruera E, Suarez-Almazor M. Opioid rotation for toxicity reduction in terminal cancer patients. J Pain Symptom Manage 1995;10:378–84.
33. Inouye SK, Charpentier PA. Precipitating factors for delirium in hospitalized elderly persons. Predictive model and interrelationship with baseline vulnerability. JAMA 1996;275:852–7.
34. Massie MJ, Holland J, Glass E. Delirium in terminally ill cancer patients. Am J Psychiatry 1983;140:1048–50.
35. Fang CK, Chen HW, Liu SI, et al. Prevalence, detection and treatment of delirium in terminal cancer inpatients: a prospective survey. Jpn J Clin Oncol 2008;38: 56–63.
36. Caraceni A, Nanni O, Maltoni M, et al. Impact of delirium on the short term prognosis of advanced cancer patients. Italian Multicenter Study Group on Palliative Care. Cancer 2000;89:1145–9.
37. Walker M, Cross H, Smith S, et al. Nonconvulsive status epilepticus: Epilepsy Research Foundation workshop reports. Epileptic Disord 2005;7:253–96.
38. Husain AM, Horn GJ, Jacobson MP. Non-convulsive status epilepticus: usefulness of clinical features in selecting patients for urgent EEG. J Neurol Neurosurg Psychiatr 2003;74:189–91.
39. Hormigo A, Liberato B, Lis E, et al. Nonconvulsive status epilepticus in patients with cancer: imaging abnormalities. Arch Neurol 2004;61:362–5.
40. Cohen N, Strauss G, Lew R, et al. Should prophylactic anticonvulsants be administered to patients with newly-diagnosed cerebral metastases? A retrospective analysis. J Clin Oncol 1988;6:1621–4.
41. van Breemen MS, Wilms EB, Vecht CJ. Epilepsy in patients with brain tumours: epidemiology, mechanisms, and management. Lancet Neurol 2007;6:421–30.
42. Glantz MJ, Cole BF, Forsyth PA, et al. Practice parameter: anticonvulsant prophylaxis in patients with newly diagnosed brain tumors. Report of the Quality Standards Subcommittee of the American Academy of Neurology. Neurology 2000;54:1886–93.
43. Hughes JR, Zak SM. EEG and clinical changes in patients with chronic seizures associated with slowly growing brain tumors. Arch Neurol 1987;44:540–3.
44. Harden CL, Huff JS, Schwartz TH, et al. Reassessment: Neuroimaging in the emergency patient presenting with seizure (an evidence-based review): report of the Therapeutics and Technology Assessment Subcommittee of the American Academy of Neurology. Neurology 2007;69:1772–80.

45. Krumholz A, Wiebe S, Gronseth G, et al. Practice parameter: evaluating an apparent unprovoked first seizure in adults (an evidence-based review): report of the Quality Standards Subcommittee of the American Academy of Neurology and the American Epilepsy Society. Neurology 2007;69:1996–2007.

46. Forsyth PA, Weaver S, Fulton D, et al. Prophylactic anticonvulsants in patients with brain tumour. Can J Neurol Sci 2003;30:106–12.

47. Engel J. Seizures and epilepsy. Philadelphia: F.A. Davis Co.; 1989.

48. Delattre JY, Safai B, Posner JB. Erythema multiforme and Stevens-Johnson syndrome in patients receiving cranial irradiation and phenytoin. Neurology 1988;38:194–8.

49. Skelton MR, Goldberg RM, O'Neil BH. A case of oxaliplatin-related posterior reversible encephalopathy syndrome. Clin Colorectal Cancer 2007;6:386–8.

50. Ozcan C, Wong SJ, Hari P. Reversible posterior leukoencephalopathy syndrome and bevacizumab. N Engl J Med 2006;354:980–2 [discussion: 2].

51. Glusker P, Recht L, Lane B. Reversible posterior leukoencephalopathy syndrome and bevacizumab. N Engl J Med 2006;354:980–2 [discussion: 2].

52. Hinchey J, Chaves C, Appignani B, et al. A reversible posterior leukoencephalopathy syndrome. N Engl J Med 1996;334:494–500.

53. Stott VL, Hurrell MA, Anderson TJ. Reversible posterior leukoencephalopathy syndrome: a misnomer reviewed. Intern Med J 2005;35:83–90.

54. Bartynski WS. Posterior reversible encephalopathy syndrome, part 1: fundamental imaging and clinical features. AJNR Am J Neuroradiol 2008;29:1036–42.

55. Graus F, Rogers LR, Posner JB. Cerebrovascular complications in patients with cancer. Medicine (Baltimore) 1985;64:16–35.

56. Perez-Lazaro C, Santos S, Morales-Rull JL, et al. Letus como primera manifestación de una neoplasia pancreática oculta [Stroke as the first manifestation of a concealed pancreatic neoplasia]. Rev Neurol 2004;38:332–5.

57. Taccone FS, Jeangette SM, Blecic SA. First-ever stroke as initial presentation of systemic cancer. J Stroke Cerebrovasc Dis 2008;17:169–74.

58. Kwon HM, Kang BS, Yoon BW. Stroke as the first manifestation of concealed cancer. J Neurol Sci 2007;258:80–3.

59. Cestari DM, Weine DM, Panageas KS, et al. Stroke in patients with cancer: incidence and etiology. Neurology 2004;62:2025–30.

60. Chaturvedi S, Ansell J, Recht L. Should cerebral ischemic events in cancer patients be considered a manifestation of hypercoagulability? Stroke 1994;25:1215–8.

61. Zhang YY, Chan DK, Cordato D, et al. Stroke risk factor, pattern and outcome in patients with cancer. Acta Neurol Scand 2006;114:378–83.

62. Kreisl TN, Toothaker T, Karimi S, et al. Ischemic stroke in patients with primary brain tumors. Neurology 2008;70:2314–20.

63. el-Shami K, Griffiths E, Streiff M. Nonbacterial thrombotic endocarditis in cancer patients: pathogenesis, diagnosis, and treatment. Oncologist 2007;12:518–23.

64. Asopa S, Patel A, Khan OA, et al. Non-bacterial thrombotic endocarditis. Eur J Cardiothorac Surg 2007;32:696–701.

65. Edoute Y, Haim N, Rinkevich D, et al. Cardiac valvular vegetations in cancer patients: a prospective echocardiographic study of 200 patients. Am J Med 1997;102:252–8.

66. Bedikian A, Valdivieso M, Luna M, et al. Nonbacterial thrombotic endocarditis in cancer patients: comparison of characteristics of patients with and without concomitant disseminated intravascular coagulation. Med Pediatr Oncol 1978;4:149–57.

67. Singhal AB, Topcuoglu MA, Buonanno FS. Acute ischemic stroke patterns in infective and nonbacterial thrombotic endocarditis: a diffusion-weighted magnetic resonance imaging study. Stroke 2002;33:1267–73.

68. Rogers LR, Cho ES, Kempin S, et al. Cerebral infarction from non-bacterial thrombotic endocarditis. Clinical and pathological study including the effects of anticoagulation. Am J Med 1987;83:746–56.

69. Smith JS, Cha S, Mayo MC, et al. Serial diffusion-weighted magnetic resonance imaging in cases of glioma: distinguishing tumor recurrence from postresection injury. J Neurosurg 2005;103:428–38.

70. Murros KE, Toole JF. The effect of radiation on carotid arteries. A review article. Arch Neurol 1989;46:449–55.

71. Bowers DC, Liu Y, Leisenring W, et al. Late-occurring stroke among long-term survivors of childhood leukemia and brain tumors: a report from the Childhood Cancer Survivor Study. J Clin Oncol 2006;24:5277–82.

72. Li SH, Chen WH, Tang Y, et al. Incidence of ischemic stroke post-chemotherapy: a retrospective review of 10,963 patients. Clin Neurol Neurosurg 2006;108: 150–6.

73. Czaykowski PM, Moore MJ, Tannock IF. High risk of vascular events in patients with urothelial transitional cell carcinoma treated with cisplatin based chemotherapy. J Urol 1998;160:2021–4.

74. Saynak M, Cosar-Alas R, Yurut-Caloglu V, et al. Chemotherapy and cerebrovascular disease. J BUON 2008;13:31–6.

75. Wall JG, Weiss RB, Norton L, et al. Arterial thrombosis associated with adjuvant chemotherapy for breast carcinoma: a Cancer and Leukemia Group B Study. Am J Med 1989;87:501–4.

76. Lefkovitz NW, Roessmann U, Kori SH. Major cerebral infarction from tumor embolus. Stroke 1986;17:555–7.

77. Klein P, Haley EC, Wooten GF, et al. Focal cerebral infarctions associated with perivascular tumor infiltrates in carcinomatous leptomeningeal metastases. Arch Neurol 1989;46:1149–52.

78. Kawanami T, Kurita K, Yamakawa M, et al. Cerebrovascular disease in acute leukemia: a clinicopathological study of 14 patients. Intern Med 2002;41: 1130–4.

79. Scaravilli FC, Cook GC. Parasitis and fungal infections. In: Graham DI, Lantos D, editors. 6th edition, Greenfield's neuropathology, vol. 2. London: Arnold; 1997. p. 543–8.

80. Poungvarin N, Bhoopat W, Viriyavejakul A, et al. Effects of dexamethasone in primary supratentorial intracerebral hemorrhage. N Engl J Med 1987;316: 1229–33.

81. Cardoso ER, Peterson EW. Pituitary apoplexy: a review. Neurosurgery 1984;14: 363–73.

82. Symon L, Mohanty S. Haemorrhage in pituitary tumours. Acta Neurochir (Wien) 1982;65:41–9.

83. Ebersold MJ, Laws ER Jr, Scheithauer BW, et al. Pituitary apoplexy treated by transsphenoidal surgery. A clinicopathological and immunocytochemical study. J Neurosurg 1983;58:315–20.

84. Biousse V, Newman NJ, Oyesiku NM. Precipitating factors in pituitary apoplexy. J Neurol Neurosurg Psychiatr 2001;71:542–5.

85. Chamberlain MC, Kormanik PA, Barba D. Complications associated with intraventricular chemotherapy in patients with leptomeningeal metastases. J Neurosurg 1997;87:694–9.

86. Olson ME, Chernik NL, Posner JB. Infiltration of the leptomeninges by systemic cancer. A clinical and pathologic study. Arch Neurol 1974;30:122–37.
87. Engelhard HH, Corsten LA. Leptomeningeal metastasis of primary central nervous system (CNS) neoplasms. Cancer Treat Res 2005;125:71–85.
88. Niermeijer JM, Somers M, Spliet W, et al. Rapidly progressive coma, hydrocephalus and leukoencephalopathy as presenting features of leptomeningeal metastases. J Neurol 2007;254:1757–8.
89. Wong ET, Joseph JT. Meningeal carcinomatosis in lung cancer. Case 1. Carcinomatous leptomeningeal metastases. J Clin Oncol 2000;18:2926–7.
90. Posner JB. Leptomeningeal metastases. In: Posner JB, editor. Neurologic complications of cancer, vol. 45. Philadelphia: F.A. Davis Co.; 1995. p. 143–71.
91. Wen P. Leptomeningeal metastases. In: Black P, Loeffler J, editors. Cancer of the nervous system. Cambridge: Blackwell Science; 1997. p. 288–309.
92. Grossman SA, Moynihan TJ. Neoplastic meningitis. Neurol Clin 1991;9:843–56.
93. Bruno MK, Raizer J. Leptomeningeal metastases from solid tumors (meningeal carcinomatosis). Cancer Treat Res 2005;125:31–52.
94. Twijnstra A, Ongerboer de Visser BW, van Zanten AP, et al. Serial lumbar and ventricular cerebrospinal fluid biochemical marker measurements in patients with leptomeningeal metastases from solid and hematological tumors. J Neurooncol 1989;7:57–63.
95. Freilich RJ, Krol G, DeAngelis LM. Neuroimaging and cerebrospinal fluid cytology in the diagnosis of leptomeningeal metastasis. Ann Neurol 1995;38:51–7.
96. Mokri B, Parisi JE, Scheithauer BW, et al. Meningeal biopsy in intracranial hypotension: meningeal enhancement on MRI. Neurology 1995;45:1801–7.
97. Rogers LR, Remer SE, Tejwani S. Durable response of breast cancer leptomeningeal metastasis to capecitabine monotherapy. Neuro Oncol 2004;6:63–4.
98. Boogerd W, Dorresteijn LD, van Der Sande JJ, et al. Response of leptomeningeal metastases from breast cancer to hormonal therapy. Neurology 2000;55:117–9.
99. Ozdogan M, Samur M, Bozcuk HS, et al. Durable remission of leptomeningeal metastasis of breast cancer with letrozole: a case report and implications of biomarkers on treatment selection. Jpn J Clin Oncol 2003;33:229–31.
100. Taillibert S, Hildebrand J. Treatment of central nervous system metastases: parenchymal, epidural, and leptomeningeal. Curr Opin Oncol 2006;18:637–43.
101. Mehta M, Bradley K. Radiation therapy for leptomeningeal cancer. Cancer Treat Res 2005;125:147–58.
102. Dalmau J, Rosenfeld MR. Paraneoplastic syndromes of the CNS. Lancet Neurol 2008;7:327–40.
103. Darnell RB, Posner JB. Paraneoplastic syndromes involving the nervous system. N Engl J Med 2003;349:1543–54.
104. Posner JB. Paraneoplastic syndromes. In: Posner JB, editor. Neurologic complications of cancer. Philadelphia: F.A. Davis Co; 1995. p. 353–84.
105. Graus F, Delattre JY, Antoine JC, et al. Recommended diagnostic criteria for paraneoplastic neurological syndromes. J Neurol Neurosurg Psychiatr 2004;75:1135–40.

Emergent Management of Malignancy-Related Acute Airway Obstruction

Pierre R. Theodore, MD

KEYWORDS

• Malignant airway obstruction • Stent • Laser • Bronchoscopy

Of the roughly 200,000 new cases of lung cancer per year in the United States, an estimated 30% will develop clinically evident endoluminal disease.[1] A fraction of these patients will go on to develop central airway obstruction. Central airway obstruction is often classified as either endoluminal, extraluminal, or mixed (**Fig. 1**). The nature of the obstruction is critical, as this often governs the use of stent versus endobronchial tumor resection or a combination of these approaches. Generally, the diagnosis of intrinsic versus extrinsic obstruction can be made only through expert bronchoscopy, although CT scanning may demonstrate likely invasion of the tracheal wall by tumor. Biopsy of critically narrowed airway processes must be undertaken with great caution, as inflammation or hemorrhage from airway manipulation can result in complete luminal ablation.[2] Definitive management involves mechanical removal of obstructing lesion in association with laser, argon beam coagulation, or electrocautery; stent placement; or ablation with radiation or photodynamic therapy (PDT). The immediate results of management of symptomatic central airway obstruction are excellent, with low procedural mortality (<5%) and improvement in the symptoms in the vast majority of patients.[3,4] Complications, such as hemorrhage, stent migration, and perforation of the airway, are uncommon. Long-term control of tumor through endobronchial techniques has also been described.[5,6]

SYMPTOMS OF AIRWAY OBSTRUCTION

Shortness of breath is often a chronic symptom associated with tumors of the lung. The presence of airway obstruction with greater than 50% stenosis of the central airways is associated with stridor and tachypnea.[3,4] Stridor occurs when erratic air currents pass through the obstructed tracheobronchial tree, resulting in high-pitch breath sounds. The effect is generally most marked on inspiration and can progress

Division of Thoracic Surgery, Department of Surgery, University of California at San Francisco, 505 Parnassus Avenue, MUW 405, San Francisco, CA 94143, USA
E-mail address: theodorep@surgery.ucsf.edu

Emerg Med Clin N Am 27 (2009) 231–241
doi:10.1016/j.emc.2009.01.009
0733-8627/09/$ – see front matter © 2009 Elsevier Inc. All rights reserved.

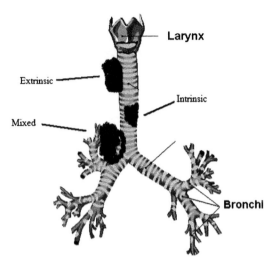

Fig. 1. Categories of central airway occlusion: Obstructions of the central tracheobronchial tree are classified as extrinsic, intrinsic, or mixed type.

to near-complete obstruction as a result of infection, inflammation, or manipulation of the airway. Malignant central airway obstruction can also produce dyspnea, hemorrhage, obstructive pneumonia, or a combination of these findings. Progressive symptoms of central airway obstruction represent a true surgical emergency. When the specialized care required for stent placement is unavailable and the patient is in jeopardy of progression to complete obstruction, fiberoptic awake intubation with a small (5–0 or 6–0 F) wire-reinforced endotracheal tube is the most expeditious means of securing the airway. Usually, a smaller tube can be guided with bronchoscopy past even the tightest of strictures. Repeated attempts of direct laryngoscopy and orotracheal intubation are to be discouraged due to the risk of inflammation and hemorrhage. Awake endotracheal intubation permits direct visualization-guided access to the airway, with minimized trauma to the upper airway. Once access beyond the obstruction is gained, the patient may be further sedated by inhalational or intravenous anesthetic agents and transferred urgently to a center with interventional pulmonary and thoracic oncology services.

EVALUATION

CT scanning of the neck and chest is the most effective initial study to assess the location and extent of the airway obstruction. For patients who can tolerate lying flat for the study, the CT (**Fig. 2**) provides the anatomic detail that permits planning of therapy. The study is assessed for location of primary tumor, the degree of intrinsic versus extrinsic compression, and the length of the stricture. Furthermore, the relationship of the narrowing of the trachea relative to the larynx or the carina is readily assessed. For bronchial lesions, the extent of postobstructive atelectasis or infection is observed.[7] Experience suggests that magnetic resonance imaging (MRI) is less useful in the assessment of central airway occlusion, with the exception of cases in which the suspected airway compromise is from large vessels (arch aneurysm, innominate artery aneurysm, or congenital vascular malformation). Flexible bronchoscopy provides a definitive view of the intraluminal disease but should be performed with

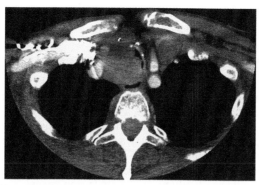

Fig. 2. CT scan of mid trachea demonstrating compression by paratracheal lymphadenopathy.

preparation for management of the airway obstruction with laser, rigid bronchoscopy, or stent placement, as described in the next section.

Rigid Bronchoscopy

Rigid bronchoscopy is an indispensable tool of the surgeon or advanced interventional pulmonologist for management of acute airway obstructive phenomena that result from tumors, foreign bodies, or hemoptysis. The rigid instrumentation required for access to the trachea and proximal airways is not tolerated by the awake patient and requires general anesthesia.[8] Furthermore, the hemodynamic alterations in heart rate and blood pressure triggered by the autonomic response to rigid bronchoscopy mandate close monitoring and management. Gas exchange with the rigid bronchoscope despite high-pressure "jet" ventilation can be poor. For these reasons, most surgeons prefer to perform rigid bronchoscopy in an OR or dedicated bronchoscopy suite with an attentive anesthesia staff. Paralytic muscle relaxant is indispensable to facilitate placement of the rigid bronchoscope into the airway. Generally, a standard endotracheal tube greater than or equal to 7.5 F is advanced into the airway to permit an unpressured evaluation of the lesion or obstructive process with flexible bronchoscopy.[8,9] It is very rare that the rigid bronchoscope is required to establish a patent airway as a first maneuver. As a practical measure, connections, light sources, and compatibility between the rigid bronchoscope and the jet ventilator should be assured before commencing the procedure. Following an initial assessment with the flexible bronchoscope in either an awake patient or via a small endotracheal tube, the rigid bronchoscope is advanced under direct vision past the vocal cords. Generally, anesthesia is induced with an IV agent coupled with a muscle relaxant, and the patient is maintained on an IV sedative infusion (ie, propofol) as the seal of the cuffless rigid bronchoscope is poor and loss of inhaled anesthetic common.

Atlantoaxial (C1–C2) subluxation is a significant concern in patients with inflammatory conditions of the spine (eg, rheumatoid arthritis) or congenital atlantoaxial ligamentous laxity (eg, Trisomy 21) and the elderly. In patients considered at high risk for cervical spine dislocation during neck extension, particular care must be exercised when introducing the rigid scope to the airway and during manipulations in the procedure. Patients and families should be apprised of the risk of spinal cord trauma in such higher-risk patients. At the conclusion of the procedure (laser ablation, mechanical coring out of lesions, or stent placement), the patient is typically reintubated with a standard endotracheal tube and weaned from the ventilator as tolerated. Several recent series have demonstrated the safety and efficacy of rigid bronchoscopy in the management of central airway occlusion from malignant disease, which is, at present, our strategy of choice for acute and emergent management.[10–12]

ND:YAG LASER THERAPY

Several large series have convincingly demonstrated the safety and efficacy of neodymium-yttrium-aluminum-garnet (Nd:YAG) laser photoradiation since its introduction in the 1980s.[13] With the principal aim of palliation, Nd:YAG laser is capable of both vaporization of obstructing tissue and providing hemostasis. With the laser set at between 20 and 50 W with 2 to 4 seconds of pulses applied to the tumor bulk, the luminal diameter can be restored following removal of any chunks of tumor remaining in the airway after laser application is complete. The laser beam is applied in a sweeping motion across the tumor's apex to lessen the risk of airway perforation. Most clinicians perform laser ablation in conjunction with rigid bronchoscopy. The rigid bronchoscope gives ready access for manual tumor debulking or tamponade of bleeding. A flexible bronchoscope can be placed through the rigid device, permitting precise guidance of the laser tip. Major morbidity and mortality associated with the use of the laser are infrequent. Perforations of the airway, hemorrhage, and respiratory failure with inability to wean from the ventilator have been described. The immediate results are generally gratifying, with the majority of patients describing improvement.[4] In cases in which urgent clearance of the airway is required, Nd:YAG laser in combination with rigid bronchoscopy provides the most immediate reestablishment of sufficient airway luminal diameter.

AIRWAY STENTING

Indications for acute placement of an airway stent[14] are summarized in **Box 1**. Airway stents provide significant benefits beyond laser fulguration alone. For central airway obstructions from intrinsic (intraluminal) lesions, an airway stent is most commonly deployed in concert with Nd:YAG sessions. Stents are classified as metallic or silicon based and covered or noncovered (**Figs. 3–7**). Virtually all current commercially available airway stents are self-expanding. However, endoluminal balloons can be of benefit in expanding tightly stenosed airways before stent deployment. Approved stents include the polymer Polyflex stent (Boston Scientific, Natick, MA) and the nitinol composite stents, such as the Ultraflex (Boston Scientific) and the Alveolus (Alveolus Inc, Charlotte, NC, USA).

The latter-generation, covered wall stents provide considerable advantages over previous uncovered stents, including less rapid in-stent stenosis and application in smaller airways.[5,15] Polyflex stents do not have studs outside, so they are more prone to migration. The thin, self-expanding wall Ultraflex (Boston Scientific) stents and Alveolus (Alveolus Inc) stents both have thin polymer membranes. Recent reports support

---

Box 1
Indications for central airway stents in the setting of malignancy

Airway obstruction from intrinsic or extrinsic compression

Supplemental therapy to laser ablation or PDT or coring out of bulky tumor to preserve patent lumen

Failure of local control with laser, PDT, or radiation therapy treatments

Treatment of tracheoesophageal fistula

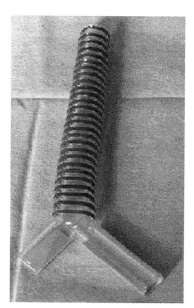

Fig. 3. Dumon Y stent tailored for right and left mainstem bronchi.

the concept that airway stenting for obstructive airway lesions results in improved quality of life, with acceptable rates of morbidity.[16] About 80% to 90% of patients with tumor-related airway stenosis have reported relief of symptoms with stent placement.[14] Airway stenting generates no consistent improvement in pulmonary function tests, but patients report improved symptoms and decreased work of breathing. These outcomes are most pronounced with treatment of tracheal lesion, and there is less benefit from addressing stenosis of mainstem bronchi.[17] If postobstructive atelectasis has persisted for more than 2 weeks, it is unlikely that stenting will achieve significant re-expansion. If the obstruction is acute, or there is greater than 50% stenosis, airway loss can be life threatening; in these cases, it is often more prudent to intubate distal to the lesion and perform therapeutic pulmonary toilet before addressing the principal stenosis. Lesions that are at risk of acute restenosis after

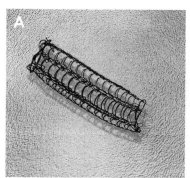
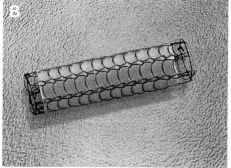

Fig. 4. Ultraflex uncovered and Ultraflex covered wall stent. (*Courtesy of* Boston Scientific, Natick, MA; with permission.)

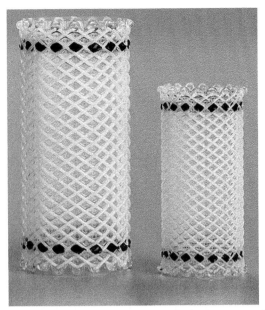

Fig. 5. Silicone-based removable covered stent (Polyflex). (*Courtesy of* Boston Scientific, Natick, MA; with permission.)

debulking or extrinsic lesions not associated with transmucosal endoluminal disease are often well managed with stent placement.[18] The only absolute contraindication to stent placement is extrinsic compression from an aneursymal vessel, as stent placement is associated with an unacceptable risk of erosion into the adjacent vessel with catastrophic hemorrhage.

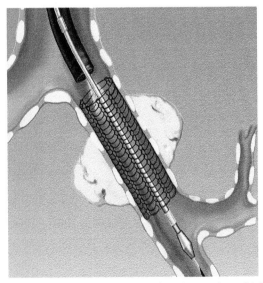

Fig. 6. Schematic representation of deployment of mainstem bronchial stent for extrinsic compressing lesion of left mainstem bronchus.

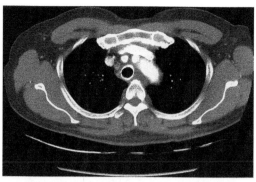

Fig. 7. CT scan demonstrating stent placed for mid-tracheal obstructing lesion with restored normal luminal diameter.

Complications of stent placement (**Table 1**) are encountered in the acute and long-term setting. The overall mortality from stent placement is very low[15] and typically related to acute loss of airway control from hemorrhage or, rarely, from an acute tear of the airway resulting in an inability to ventilate the patient. Laser ablation and coring out of lesions via rigid bronchoscopy before stent placement can be associated with hemorrhage in the short term. Although early complications are uncommon, longer-term complications from stent placement are common (see **Table 1**) and include migration, infection, or granulomatous tissue, further compromising the luminal diameter. Mechanical insufficiencies of the stents have been reported.[15] Granulation tissue encroaching on the lumen can often be managed with repeated laser ablation and balloon dilation.

TRACHEOSTOMY WITH WIRE-REINFORCED LONG-LENGTH PROSTHESIS

Several commercial tracheotomy prostheses are available (Smith Medical, Cook), which are of long or adjustable length (up to 18 cm), permitting passage of a secure airway past tracheal obstructions and can be indispensable in urgent situations. The prostheses (ie, "Bivona tubes") are often wire reinforced to resist the radial compressive force of luminal tumor or paratracheal mass. The long-segment tubes can be placed even in awake, sedated patients with adequate local anesthetic followed by tracheostomy and expeditious bronchoscopic guidance past tracheal obstruction. This provides a stable patent airway that permits a spontaneously breathing nonsedated patient to be managed definitively at a later time. Adjustable prostheses (**Fig. 8**) are particularly useful, as the length can be tailored to terminate just above

Table 1
Complications of stent placement

Immediate	Stent-Related Complications	Long Term
Malposition with deployment	Stent fracture or fatigue	Infection and increased respiratory secretion retention
Perforation of airway	Erosion through airway	Granulation tissue
Airway obstruction or aspiration	Migration after therapy for tumor mass	Tumor progression and luminal obstruction

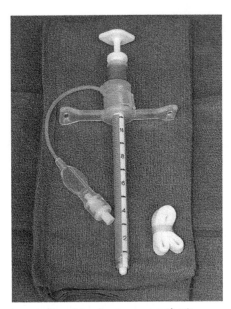

Fig. 8. "Bivona" stent–wire-reinforced tracheotomy prosthesis.

the carina. This approach provides adequate luminal diameter (6–8 F) until more definitive therapy, such as external beam irradiation or indwelling, tracheal stent placement, can be performed. Long tracheostomy prostheses are limited in application to stenosis of the trachea. The availability of these prostheses can permit emergent stabilization of an impending airway occlusion.

EXTERNAL BEAM RADIATION THERAPY, HIGH-DOSE ENDOBRONCHIAL BRACHYTHERAPY, AND PHOTODYNAMIC THERAPY

Several less invasive modalities have been adopted recently for management of tumors obstructing the central airways. The principal issue is that each of these modalities require longer time frames for effect and are often best used in conjunction with mechanical (or laser) debulking maneuvers to immediately resolve obstruction.

High-dose endobronchial brachytherapy in conjunction with other modalities appears to be an effective approach to unresectable disease and may provide an important adjunct to endoluminal laser ablative therapies. Since Speiser and Spratling reported their series of over 250 patients treated with endobronchial radiation therapy, demonstrating a 60% to 90% rate of response, enthusiasm has increased for intraluminal radiation.[19,20] This option, however, has a 15% risk of major complication, including radiation-induced pneumonitis and major hemorrhage.[21] Endobronchial brachytherapy Iridium 192 has shown promise in reducing the complications of direct interstitial implantation of radioactive seeds. The response rate is high, with good symptomatic improvement and radiographic resolution of postobstructive atelectasis. The response is durable, with most lesions not showing local recurrence within 6 months after completion of therapy.[21] Although the response rate is high, the use of endobronchial radiation therapy alone in the setting of acute airway obstruction by malignancy is inappropriate. A combination of laser fulguration of tumor and endobronchial irradiation permits immediate relief of obstruction in addition to a measure of local control of tumor.

PDT

PDT uses a photosensitizing agent (photofrin), which, when administered intravenously, is selectively retained within tumor cells. The agents are activated on exposure to a light of proper wavelength generating cytotoxic oxygen radicals, which lead to tumor necrosis. PDT has been used for obstructing lesions of the central airways that are not at immediate risk of airway occlusion.[22] PDT allows for satisfactory local control of submucosal isolated tumors of the airway in patients who are poor candidates for surgery. In addition to the laser and rigid bronchoscopic relief of airway obstruction, PDT as an adjunct can prevent or delay reocclusion.

EXTERNAL BEAM RADIATION THERAPY AND MULTIMODAL THERAPY

Two recently completed studies[23,24] of external beam irradiation or brachytherapy in conjunction with Nd:YAG laser for patients with central airway occlusion from malignancy demonstrated improved median survival versus Nd:YAG therapy alone. The result suggests that combination therapy at a center experienced in both endobronchial techniques and thoracic radiation oncology can achieve improved rates of local control and survival. Tumor debulking can be carried out mechanically by the blade of the rigid bronchoscope in combination with Nd:YAG laser for hemostasis. Brachytherapy is delayed for 2 to 4 weeks after laser debulking and consists of 3 afterloading sessions at weekly intervals, performed with an endobronchial irradiation dose of 5 Gy per session.[23] This approach has the advantage of both addressing the airway obstruction and improving disease-free survival.

SUMMARY

Central airway occlusion occurs in roughly a third of all patients with intrathoracic malignancies and is a significant source of morbidity and poor quality of life. The symptoms of stridor, shortness of breath, and limitation of physical exertion are indications for palliative maneuvers and procedures. The urgency of the clinical scenario dictates the approach to the disease. In patients with stable airways, CT scanning and, occasionally, MRI permit careful planning, such as type and length of stent or the feasibility of external beam irradiation. Flexible bronchoscopy can permit the most careful evaluation of the airway, but definitive therapy should be planned to limit the number of manipulations of the tenuous airway. For patients presenting with acute life-threatening central airway occlusion, obtaining a secure airway expeditiously remains the cornerstone of management. Such patients should be offered intubation in a controlled setting (the OR being ideal) with available rigid bronchoscopy. Manual coring out of the airway lesion and placement of a secure endotracheal tube are the most rapid means of restoring a satisfactory lumen. In patients who have a sufficient luminal diameter and intrinsic tumor, Nd:YAG laser is the approach of choice to vaporize and reduce the obstruction. For incompletely resolved airway obstructions or those at high risk for recurrence, stent placement, particularly self-expanding metal stents, are an effective means of maintaining patency despite the adverse events sometimes encountered. Endoluminal high dose radiation therapy and brachytherapy have the additional benefit of treatment of tumor with potential longer-term local control and should be considered in consultation with radiation oncology colleagues. Although long-term outcomes of patients with malignancy-related airway obstruction are poor, the majority (80%) will have symptoms significantly improved by surgery. This improvement related to quality of life provides the rationale for thorough, thoughtful management of central airway obstruction.

REFERENCES

1. Stohr S, Bolliger CT. Stents in the management of malignant airway obstruction. Monaldi Arch Chest Dis 1999;54:264–8.
2. Wood DE. Airway stenting. Chest Surg Clin N Am 2001;11:841–60.
3. Ernst A, Feller-Kopman D, Becker HD, et al. Central airway obstruction. Am J Respir Crit Care Med 2004;169:1278–97.
4. Amjadi K, Voduc N, Cruysberghs, et al. Impact of interventional bronchoscopy on quality of life in malignant airway obstruction. Respiration 2008 Aug 30 [Epub ahead of print].
5. Noppen M, Poppe K, D'Haese J, et al. Interventional bronchoscopy for treatment of tracheal obstruction secondary to benign or malignant thyroid disease. Chest 2004;125(2):723–30.
6. Moghissi K, Dixon K, Thorpe JA, et al. Photodynamic therapy (PDT) in early central lung cancer: a treatment option for patients ineligible for surgical resection. Thorax 2007;62(5):391–5.
7. Zarić B, Canak V, Sarcev T, et al. Interventional pulmonology techniques for immediate desobstruction of malignant central airway obstruction. J BUON 2007;12(1):11–22.
8. Purugganan RV. Intravenous anesthesia for thoracic procedures. Curr Opin Anaesthesiol 2008;21(1):1–7.
9. Breitenbücher A, Chhajed PN, Brutsche MH, et al. Long-term follow-up and survival after Ultraflex stent insertion in the management of complex malignant airway stenosis. Respiration 2008;75(4):443–9.
10. Moghissi K, Dixon K. Bronchoscopic Nd:YAG laser treatment in lung cancer, 30 years on: an institutional review. Lasers Med Sci 2006;21(4):186–91.
11. Jeon K, Kim H, Yu CM, et al. Rigid bronchoscopic intervention in patients with respiratory failure caused by malignant central airway obstruction. J Thorac Oncol 2006;1(4):319–23.
12. Stephens KE Jr, Wood DE. Bronchoscopic management of central airway obstruction. J Thorac Cardiovasc Surg 2000;119(2):289–96.
13. Personne C, Colchen A, Leroy M, et al. Indications and technique for endoscopic laser resections in bronchology. A critical analysis based upon 2,284 resections. J Thorac Cardiovasc Surg 1986;91(5):710–5.
14. Wood DE, Liu YH, Vallières E, et al. Airway stenting for malignant and benign tracheobronchial stenosis. Ann Thorac Surg 2003;76(1):167–74.
15. Colt HG, Dumon JF. Airway stents. Present and future. Clin Chest Med 1995;16(3):465–78.
16. Han CC, Prasetyo D, Wright GM. Endobronchial palliation using Nd:YAG laser is associated with improved survival when combined with multimodal adjuvant treatments. J Thorac Oncol 2007;2(1):59–64.
17. Miyazawa T, Miyazu Y, Iwamoto Y, et al. Stenting at the flow-limiting segment in tracheobronchial stenosis due to lung cancer. Am J Respir Crit Care Med 2004;169(10):1096–102.
18. Folch E, Mehta AC. Airway interventions in the tracheobronchial tree. Semin Respir Crit Care Med 2008;29(4):441–52.
19. Speiser B, Spratling L. Intraluminal bronchial radiation technique: complications and results in 250 patients. In: Nori D, editor. Proceedings of the international conference in thoracic oncology and brachytherapy. New York: Nucletron; 1991. p. 96–8.

20. Nag S, Abitbol AA, Anderson LL, et al. Consensus guidelines for high dose rate remote brachytherapy in cervical, endometrial, and endobronchial tumors. Clinical Research Committee, American Endocurietherapy Society. Int J Radiat Oncol Biol Phys 1993;27(5):1241–4.
21. Nori D, Allison R, Kaplan B, et al. High dose-rate intraluminal irradiation in bronchogenic carcinoma. Technique and results. Chest 1993;104(4):1006–11.
22. Loewen GM, Pandey R, Bellnier D, et al. Endobronchial photodynamic therapy for lung cancer. Lasers Surg Med 2006;38(5):364–70.
23. Canak V, Zarić B, Milovancev A, et al. Combination of interventional pulmonology techniques (Nd:YAG laser resection and brachytherapy) with external beam radiotherapy in the treatment of lung cancer patients with Karnofsky Index < or =50. J BUON 2006;11(4):447–56.
24. Mallick I, Sharma S, Behera D. Endobronchial brachytherapy for symptom palliation in non-small cell lung cancer - Analysis of symptom response, endoscopic improvement and quality of life. Lung Cancer 2006;55(3):313–8.

Superior Vena Cava Syndrome

Jonathan F. Wan, BASc, MD, FRCPC[a,b,*], Andrea Bezjak, MD, MSc, FRCPC[a]

KEYWORDS

- Superior vena cava syndrome • Cancer
- Superior vena cava obstruction • Radiation therapy
- Endovascular stenting • Chemotherapy

Superior vena cava syndrome (SVCS) is a common complication of malignancy, especially of lung cancer and lymphoma. The frequency of SVCS varies depending on the specific malignancy. Approximately 2% to 4% of all patients with lung cancer develop SVCS at some time during their disease course.[1–6] The incidence is higher in small cell lung cancer (SCLC), given its predilection for mediastinal involvement and rapid growth; the incidence approaches 10%.[5,7,8] SVCS develops in approximately 2% to 4% of non-Hodgkin's lymphoma (NHL)[1,4] but is relatively rare in Hodgkin's lymphoma despite the presence of mediastinal lymphadenopathy.[9] For primary mediastinal large B-cell lymphomas with sclerosis, the incidence has been reported as high as 57% in one series of 30 patients.[10] Together, lung cancer and lymphoma are responsible for over 90% of malignant causes of SVCS.[3,11] In the modern era, 60% to 90% of cases of SVCS are caused by malignant tumors, with the remaining cases accounted for largely by fibrosing mediastinitis and thrombosis of indwelling central venous devices and/or pacemaker leads.[3,12–14] The focus of this article is on the management of malignant causes of SVCS.

ANATOMY AND PHYSIOLOGY

The superior vena cava (SVC) is the major vessel collecting venous return to the heart from the head, arms, and upper torso. Compression of the SVC in malignancy is usually due to extrinsic masses in the middle or anterior mediastinum, right paratracheal or precarinal lymph node stations, and tumors extending from the right upper

Statement regarding funding/support: Dr. Wan received support from the Radiation Oncology Fellowship Program at the Princess Margaret Hospital, University of Toronto.

[a] Department of Radiation Oncology, University of Toronto, Princess Margaret Hospital, 610 University Avenue, Toronto, Ontario, Canada M5G 2M9

[b] Department of Radiation Oncology, McGill University, Montreal General Hospital, 1650 Cedar Avenue, Montreal, Quebec, Canada H3G 1A4

* Corresponding author. Department of Radiation Oncology, University of Toronto, Princess Margaret Hospital, 610 University Avenue, Toronto, Ontario, Canada M5G 2M9.
E-mail address: jonathan.wan@muhc.mcgill.ca (J.F. Wan).

lobe bronchus. As the tumors increase in size and produce compression of the SVC, there is increased resistance to venous blood flow, which is then diverted through collateral networks that may develop. Collateral vessels that are commonly found include azygos, intercostal, mediastinal, paravertebral, hemiazygos, thoracoepigastric, internal mammary, thoracoacromioclavicular, and anterior chest wall veins.[15] The severity of SVCS is worse if the level of obstruction is below the azygos vein, underscoring the importance of this vessel in providing an alternate route for blood flow.[16] The severity of the obstruction is also dependent on the rapidity of onset of the obstruction. Collateral vessels often take several weeks to dilate sufficiently to accommodate the diverted blood flow of the SVC. The presence of collateral vessels with compression of SVC on computed tomography (CT) is a reliable indicator of the presence of SVCS with a sensitivity of 96% and specificity of 92%.[17]

PRESENTATION

Patients often complain of a variety of symptoms. The most common of these are facial or neck swelling (82%), arm swelling (68%), dyspnea (66%), cough (50%), and dilated chest veins (38%).[11,13] Patients may also report chest pain, dysphagia, hoarseness, headache, confusion, dizziness, and syncope. Orthopnea is commonly noted, since a supine position will increase the amount of blood flow to the upper torso. Attention should be given to the duration of symptoms, previous diagnosis of malignancy, or previous intravascular procedures for clues to the etiology of the syndrome. In most cases, symptoms develop over the course of several weeks allowing for collateral circulations to develop.

Worrisome signs include stridor, as this is usually indicative of laryngeal edema, as well as confusion and obtundation, since these may indicate cerebral edema. Although SVCS is now known not to be a major threat to life in most clinical scenarios, evidence of respiratory and neurologic compromise can be associated with serious or fatal outcomes. In addition, patients may have other cancer-related symptoms, such as extrinsic compression of major airway by tumor (which may be an alternate explanation for the stridor), hemoptysis, or thrombosis associated with malignant SVCS, which may need to be addressed urgently and may be more life threatening. Patients may also have B symptoms (eg, drenching night sweats, weight loss, or fevers usually associated with lymphomas) or other constitutional symptoms.

In the past, SVCS was considered to be a medical emergency. However, multiple retrospective reviews have shown that this is not the case in the absence of laryngeal/bronchial or cerebral edema.[13,14,18] Accurate diagnosis via imaging and biopsy should be obtained, since treatment approaches can vary widely depending on the histology of the malignancy. Staging investigations should be completed before initiating treatment if possible, because a decision will need to be made regarding a definitive curative approach as opposed to a palliative course of treatment.

Although no standardized grading system exists for the evaluation of SVCS, the group from Yale University have recently proposed a classification system for grading the severity of SVCS[19] as asymptomatic (grade 0), mild (grade 1), moderate (grade 2), severe (grade 3), life-threatening (grade 4), or fatal (grade 5). Cerebral edema, laryngeal edema, stridor, and hemodynamic compromise would constitute grade 3 (if mild/moderate) or grade 4 (if significant) SVCS. The authors recommend more urgent treatment be initiated in the presence of grade 3 or 4 symptoms. The proposed system has not been validated but does provide a rational framework of how to approach and triage these patients.

The diagnosis of SVCS is made on the basis of clinical signs and symptoms and confirmed by imaging studies.

EVALUATION

Physical examination should document the extent of facial, neck, and/or arm swelling, elevation of neck veins, the extent of collateral veins on the chest, and any evidence of respiratory compromise. Facial swelling and plethora are typically exacerbated when patient is supine; the resultant cyanosis can be quite dramatic. Particular attention should be given to any palpable nodes, as they may provide an easily accessible site for tissue biopsy. Routine blood work should be obtained, including complete blood counts, renal function, and liver enzymes. Abnormalities in blood work may indicate other possible sites of biopsy, such as bone marrow or liver lesions, and may influence the subsequent therapy.

Imaging Studies

The majority of patients will have an abnormal chest radiograph (84%), with the most common findings being mediastinal widening (64%) and pleural effusion (26%).[12] **Fig. 1** is an example of a chest radiograph from a patient with SVCS. The most useful imaging study is computed tomography (CT) of the chest with contrast (needed to evaluate the SVC).[20,21] CT imaging allows the level and extent of the blockage to be defined as well as an evaluation of collateral pathways of drainage. It also permits identification of the cause of the obstruction, since a malignant mass is responsible for up to 90% of SVCS. Common findings on CT include enlarged paratracheal lymph nodes with or without additional lung or pleural abnormalities. A classic example of SVCS is shown in **Fig. 2**, where contrast clearly delineates compression of the SVC and the development of collateral vessels.

Venography is primarily used if an interventional stent is planned. Radionuclide Tc-99 m venography fails to provide the diagnostic information that is supplied by chest CT regarding location and characteristics of extrinsic masses. However, this technique can be useful for identifying thrombotic obstructions within the SVC.[22,23] Magnetic resonance imaging may be useful for patients who cannot tolerate CT contrast for any reason to assess mediastinal veins.[24,25]

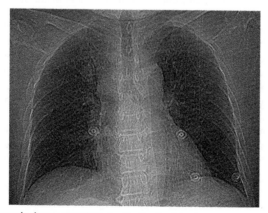

Fig. 1. Chest radiograph demonstrating mediastinal widening.

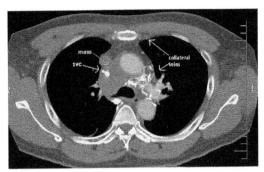

Fig. 2. Axial image of CT thorax, demonstrating a right paratracheal soft tissue mass causing narrowing and compression of SVC and presence of collaterals.

In addition to imaging of the chest, a full diagnostic workup for the suspected cancer may be appropriate either at this time or after the tissue diagnosis is obtained. For lung cancer, this typically includes imaging of the abdomen, brain, and bone; for lymphomas, this includes imaging of the abdomen and pelvis, possibly a bone marrow biopsy and a gallium and/or fluorodeoxyglucose positron emission tomographic scan, if appropriate.

Diagnostic Interventions

A tissue diagnosis is necessary to confirm the presence of a malignancy. In the absence of acute airway compromise or progressive neurologic decline from cerebral edema, initiation of therapy before obtaining a diagnosis is unwarranted given only infrequent reports of mortality from SVCS in multiple series.[13,14,18] However, the diagnostic workup should be expedited as patients may deteriorate quickly if collateral vessels are not well established. The importance of a proper diagnosis and staging of the patient cannot be overstressed. The treatment approaches vary widely depending on the type of malignancy present and whether an attempt will be made at definitive curative treatment as opposed to palliative approaches. Interventions such as radiation, chemotherapy, and/or steroids may obscure a histologic diagnosis at a later date. Radiation in particular can obscure a diagnosis in up to 42% of biopsy specimens obtained from the irradiated area after treatment.[26]

Careful clinical assessment of peripheral sites, such as supraclavicular nodes, that are easily accessible must be made before proceeding to more invasive procedures, such as bronchoscopy, mediastinoscopy, or endobronchial ultrasound guided biopsies (EBUS). Pleural effusions are also commonly found and are often accessible to thoracocentesis, although the diagnostic yield may be suboptimal.[27] Bronchoscopy has a diagnostic yield of 50% to 70% (depending on the presence of a centrally located lung mass), and transthoracic needle aspiration has a yield of 75%, whereas mediastinoscopy has a diagnostic yield of 90% to 100% in determining the cause of SVCS.[28–32] The risks associated with mediastinoscopy, predominantly bleeding and infection, are in the order of 0% to 7% in selected series.[28,29,31,33,34] No specific data exist with regard to the use of EBUS in obtaining a diagnosis in patients with SVCS, although randomized data suggest that EBUS is superior to conventional transbronchial needle aspiration in obtaining a diagnosis should mediastinoscopy be unavailable.[8,35]

MANAGEMENT

Management of superior cava syndrome due to malignancy depends on the etiology of the cancer, the extent of the disease, the severity of symptoms, and the prognosis of the patient.[19] Median life expectancy in patients with SVCS is approximately 6 months with a range of 1.5 to 9.5 months; however, estimates vary widely and are dependent on the underlying malignant condition.[36] Intervention needs to consider both treatment of the cancer and relief of the symptoms of the obstruction. Treatment of the cancer may be directed with curative intent or for palliation of symptoms alone. The intent of treatment is not always immediately clear, and therapy may need to be initiated before a full staging workup. For these reasons, the physician may wish to allow for a flexible treatment approach that would allow for conversion from a palliative approach to definitive management of the disease as the patient's status improves.

Data from randomized trials are scarce, and most evidence guiding treatment decisions are from case series. The treatment options include supportive measures, RT, chemotherapy, and stent insertion. Surgery is virtually never an option, as the presence of SVCS almost always signifies unresectable tumor within the mediastinum. Although there may be a role for surgery after induction treatment for selected patients with mediastinal nodal disease from lung cancer, it would be unlikely that a patient who presented with SVCS would have potentially resectable nodal disease. However, if in doubt, surgical input as part of multidisciplinary assessment may be sought, although the most efficient approach would be to refer to a specialist who is most likely to initiate appropriate therapy for the patient.

Interventions for Symptom Relief

Initial interventions should be directed toward supportive care and medical management. Although there are no data documenting the effectiveness of such maneuvers, these measures can be performed with minimal risk and may provide initial relief of the symptoms of SVCS. Oxygen support and attempts to minimize the hydrostatic pressure in the upper torso, such as fluid limitation, head elevation, and diuretics, may be useful in reducing symptoms in the short term.

Recognition of life-threatening symptoms suggestive of airway compromise and/or cerebral edema is essential. Evidence of severe airway compromise, such as stridor, accompanied by findings of laryngeal edema or tracheal obstruction on CT should be addressed emergently with interventions to protect the airway, such as an endotracheal tube. Management of cerebral edema associated with SVCS has not been described in the literature. Standard resuscitation techniques should be considered, such as head elevation, hyperventilation, and use of osmotic diuretics such as mannitol, if the patient presents with symptoms suggestive of cerebral edema. Imaging for an intracranial cause of cerebral edema should be obtained as well. In both cases, the patient should be hospitalized, monitored closely, and treated urgently to relieve the SVCS.

Steroids are often used as a temporary measure to reduce edema and associated symptoms,[37] but there is an absence of data documenting the effectiveness and dose of steroids in this setting. There is also a risk of obscuring the tissue diagnosis, especially if lymphoma is suspected.[3,5] In one retrospective review of 107 patients, the use of steroids and diuretics or neither therapy had a similar rate of clinical improvement of 84%.[13] However, in a symptomatic patient in whom airway edema is believed to contribute to the symptoms, steroids can be an effective intervention. No standard dosing or guidelines exist with regard to the dose of steroids to be used. At our institution, dexamethasone 4 mg orally twice a day or 4 mg orally four times a day is often initiated.

It should be emphasized that steroids should only be used as an initial temporizing measure. Chronic use of high doses of steroids can result in significant side effects, including facial swelling (cushingoid facies), and promote fluid retention, both of which could aggravate the symptoms of SVCS.[38,39] Prolonged use of high doses of cortico-steroids can also complicate assessment of therapeutic effectiveness, as the side effects of steroids can overlap with the symptoms of SVCS.

One should also be acutely aware that thrombosis may contribute to the severity of the SVCS as well as pose a major threat to life should pulmonary embolus or further thrombotic events occur. The incidence of thromboembolic events in patients with malignant SVCS has been reported as high as 38% in a group of prospectively followed patients.[40] There are less data guiding the decision to anticoagulate patients with malignant SVCS (without documented thrombus), with only an older, small, randomized trial that showed no difference in survival between patients anticoagulated versus those who were not.[41] Unfortunately, this trial did not report the incidence of pulmonary embolism. In summary, there is no evidence to support routine anticoagulation in patients with malignant SVCS in the absence of thrombosis. It appears reasonable to anticoagulate patients with demonstrable thrombus on imaging.

After a tissue diagnosis has been obtained and the extent of the disease has been determined, a decision should be made to address control of the malignant process in either a curative fashion or palliatively. Radiation, chemotherapy, or stent placement, or a combination of these modalities will play a role as the definitive intervention of SVCS, depending on the sensitivity of the specific tumor.

Radiation

Radiotherapy (RT) is an effective modality in the treatment of SVCS due to malignancy. A systemic review of the literature, conducted by Rowell and Gleeson,[5] documented that radiation was effective at providing overall relief in approximately three-quarters of SVCS due to SCLC and in two-thirds of SVCS due to non-small cell lung cancer (NSCLC).

The rapidity of response is in the range of 7 to 15 days but may be seen as early as 72 hours after initiation of therapy.[6,42–45] Relative contraindications to RT include previous treatment with radiation in the same region, certain connective tissue disorders such as scleroderma, and known radioresistant tumor types (eg, sarcoma). Response rates in the literature are often clinical, and there can be a significant discordance with objective response rates as measured by imaging. In one report, evaluation with serial venography documented complete relief in 31% and partial relief in 23% for a total objective response rate of 54%, which is somewhat lower than clinically reported response rates.[46]

The radiation treatment plan can vary based on the histology of the tumor as well as the intent of treatment. For example, a definitive course of radiation for SCLC can involve 3 to 6 weeks of daily or twice-a-day treatments (eg, 40 Gy in 15 daily fractions, 50 Gy in 25 fractions, 60 Gy in 30 fractions, or 45 Gy at fraction sizes of 1.5 Gy twice a day over 3 weeks). In NSCLC, definitive treatment takes 6 to 7 weeks to administer in daily fractions of 2 Gy. Palliative treatments are typically administered over a course of 1 to 2 weeks with larger fraction sizes of 3 Gy to 5 Gy (eg, 20 Gy in 5 fractions, 30 Gy in 10 fractions), with the goal of achieving a more rapid response by using larger daily doses. Abbreviated treatments of 2 6-Gy fractions (12 Gy/2 fractions) have been reported to be effective in older patients with poorer performance status.[47]

Radiation treatment planning usually involves CT-based simulation for designing RT fields. The fields should encompass the gross tumor volume and involved nodal regions and attempt to shield involved normal organs in the proximity of the tumor, particularly lung and esophagus, to minimize the risk of side effects. The size and configuration of the fields may be altered during the treatment course, as patients may improve symptomatically, and tumor may shrink to allow for a higher curative dose to be delivered.

Careful assessment of the patient is needed during the radiation treatment to monitor for side effects as well as progression of radioresistant tumors necessitating alternative interventions, such as stent placement and/or a protective airway if symptoms worsen. Occasionally, worsening of symptoms can be due to development of a thrombus, in which case vascular imaging and anticoagulation should be considered.

Chemotherapy

Lymphomas, SCLCs, and germ cell tumors are widely regarded as chemotherapy-sensitive tumors, with high rates of response and quick onset of tumor shrinkage. Thus, chemotherapy is often used as the initial treatment for SVCS from such tumors. RT alone can be used and can provide prompt responses as well for these malignancies; but it usually yields poorer long-term results and is used only in patients who are not candidates for chemotherapy.[4,6] Chemotherapy can relieve the symptoms of SVCS in up to 80% of patients with NHL and 77% with SCLS.[4,5] The response rate of relief from SVCS treated with chemotherapy is similar to that of RT and ranges from 7 to 15 days.[36] **Fig. 3** demonstrates the response of a patient with a chemotherapy-sensitive tumor. After several cycles of chemotherapy, the patient recovered patency of his SVC with good symptomatic relief and reduction in tumor burden.

The addition of RT to chemotherapy did not significantly affect the relief of SVCS or relapse rates in 2 randomized trials of SCLC and NSCLC as well as in a systemic review of the published data.[5,8,48] Once the symptomatic benefit is obtained, the patient may be a candidate for curative treatment, which in cases of limited-stage SCLC or early stage NHL would include the addition of RT to systemic chemotherapy, as this has been shown to decrease local recurrence rates and improve survival in these clinical scenarios.

Endovascular Stenting

Endovascular stenting can provide rapid relief by restoring venous return in patients with SVCS. Relief can be immediate, but in most series, it is reported within 24 to

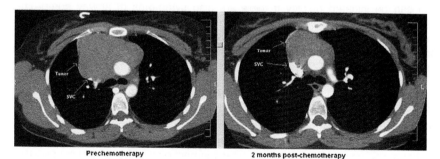

Prechemotherapy   2 months post-chemotherapy

Fig. 3. Radiographic response of patient with malignant SVCS from a chemotherapy-sensitive tumor.

72 hours following the procedure.[5,49–51] Stent placement can be especially useful when urgent intervention is indicated for patients without a tissue diagnosis or who have previously been treated with RT or in those who have known chemotherapy- and radiation-resistant tumors. In addition, endovascular stenting may be considered as a first-line intervention in patients with SVCS.[52–54] Stents provide relief from the obstruction in an immediate and direct fashion, but they do not deal with the cancer itself. Thus, in many cases, stent placement is followed by other treatments, such as radiation and/or chemotherapy.

Stent placement is usually performed under local anesthesia in an angiography suite, with introduction of a guide wire via either the subclavian or internal jugular vein with or without balloon angioplasty followed by deployment of a stent.[53,55,56] If a clot is encountered, thrombolytics are often used, although their benefit in this context remains unclear, and the morbidity of stent placement does appear higher with the use of thrombolytics.[32,36,57] Even in the absence of a visible thrombus, some advocate use of prophylactic anticoagulation (eg, with low-molecular-weight heparin) after stent placement, given the presence of a foreign body and the fact that cancer patients (particularly lung cancer patients) are at an increased risk of thrombosis. Whether this is clearly beneficial is not known. The use of steroids is also not mentioned in most studies.[36] Whether or not a particular type of stent is advantageous remains unknown.[58,59]

There are no randomized, controlled trials comparing the efficacy of endovascular stenting with radiation or chemotherapy. The most extensive data come from a systemic review of the literature by Rowell and Gleeson in which 23 stent studies were combined for a total of 159 patients with SVCS due to either SCLC or NSCLC.[36] The results were not reported separately for the different histologies. About 95% of the patients experienced complete or partial relief of their symptoms following stenting; the relapse rate was reported as 11%. In comparison, relief rates in 487 patients with SCLC treated with chemotherapy alone, chemoradiotherapy, or RT were 77%, 83%, and 78% respectively; however, in NSCLC, relief rates in 243 patients treated with chemotherapy or RT were 59% and 63%, respectively.[36] From this review, stenting appears to be the most effective and rapid treatment available to patients with SVCS due to malignancy. However, there are far fewer patients treated with stents in the literature, and patient selection may have played a role. Thus, comparison of outcomes is limited due to the absence of randomized studies. Obtaining randomized data for a direct comparison is difficult for a number of reasons: one treatment may be more immediately available than the other (eg, there may not be stent expertise, or radiation may not be immediately available), or there may be a clinical reason to favor one over the other (eg, stent may be preferred in a previous irradiated chest area; radiation can be initiated quickly if there are also symptoms of airway compromise; chemotherapy may be chosen if it is a chemosensitive tumor).[60] Thus, although randomized trials have been attempted, to date, they have not been successfully completed.[60] Whether endovascular stenting is truly superior in longer-term palliation of the symptoms of SVCS remains unknown.

SUMMARY AND RECOMMENDATIONS

SVCS is a common complication of malignancies such as lung cancer or lymphoma. The presentation is often clinically striking, especially if not recognized early enough. It requires a workup and formulation of a management plan, although not necessarily an emergency intervention. In most cases, the initial management of this syndrome should be directed at supportive care, including such maneuvers as elevation of the

Table 1
Advantages and disadvantages of radiation therapy, stent insertion, and chemotherapy

Radiation		Stent		Chemotherapy	
Advantages	*Disadvantages*	*Advantages*	*Disadvantages*	*Advantages*	*Disadvantages*
Noninvasive intervention	Symptom relief in 7–15 d	Rapid relief of symptoms usually within 24–72 h	Invasive intervention	Noninvasive intervention	Symptom relief in 7–15 d
Treats underlying malignancy	May compromise a tissue diagnosis if not yet obtained	Does not compromise a tissue diagnosis	Bleeding complications	Treats underlying malignancy	May compromise a tissue diagnosis if not yet obtained
—	May initially worsen symptoms due to inflammation	Allows option for further treatment with chemotherapy, radiation, or combined-modality therapy	Increased risk of thrombosis due to foreign object	Does not require specialized equipment	Patient may be too sick to tolerate chemotherapy
—	—	—	Does not treat the underlying malignancy	Ability to be administered in ICU	Hematologic and other toxicity

The interventions are supported by level of evidence B; there is no level A evidence specific to the management of SVCS.
Abbreviation: ICU, intensive care unit.

head, oxygen support, diuretics, and possibly steroids, although none has been proven to be of benefit. This should be followed by confirmation of the presence of venous obstruction with imaging and interventions to establish the etiology. A histologic diagnosis confirming malignancy should be obtained before initiating therapy in a patient with no previous diagnosis of cancer. Steroids are often used to decrease swelling but may obscure a histologic diagnosis. In patients with life-threatening signs, such as worsening laryngeal edema and stridorous symptoms, initial placement of an intravascular stent can provide rapid relief without compromising future treatments or diagnostic interventions. One should also be vigilant for the presence or development of thrombosis in these patients. There are no data to support routine anticoagulation in patients with malignant SVCS without evidence of thrombus.

Following a diagnosis of malignancy, a decision should be made as to whether the intent of treatment will be curative or palliative. Treatment planning should be multidisciplinary and include medical and radiation oncologists at an early stage. Treatment options include stent placement, radiation alone, chemotherapy alone, and combined-modality therapy. No randomized studies have shown superiority of one approach over the other, and the choice should be tailored to the particular clinical scenario.

For patients with a newly diagnosed chemotherapy- sensitive malignancy, such as SCLC, NHL, and germ cell tumors, systemic chemotherapy as an initial intervention is reasonable. The use of stents in severely symptomatic patients can provide rapid relief if necessary. Radiation alone is also an effective intervention in these malignancies should chemotherapy be unavailable or contraindicated.

For patients with a newly diagnosed NSCLC, endovascular stent placement or RT is recommended as a first intervention. RT may be used alone or as part of a combined-modality approach with concurrent or sequential chemotherapy. A direct comparison of RT and stent placement has not been made in a randomized, control setting, but it appears from retrospective reports that stent placement is at least as effective as radiation with regard to relief rates and is certainly more rapid. A qualitative comparison of the 3 interventions is presented in **Table 1**.

For patients who have recurrent or progressive malignancies and symptomatic SVC who have had previous radiation in the mediastinum, we recommend consideration of endovascular stents for relief of symptoms. Whether or not radiation can be delivered to the same area again will depend on the dose and technique of previous radiation. If previous RT was administered with palliative intent, ie, lower to moderate doses, further RT may be possible, but would require careful planning to avoid organs at risk of re-irradiation, particularly the spinal cord, if treated before. If previous RT was high dose, it may not be possible to safely deliver further RT, and stent would indeed be the best consideration.

For patients who are treated with radiation with severe airway obstruction, a short course of steroids (dexamethasone 4 mg orally twice a day to 4 mg orally four times a day) is reasonable during the radiation to prevent further compromise due to worsening swelling caused by acute radiation response, but there is no evidence supporting this intervention.

The treatment of SVCS secondary to malignancy must be individualized, based on previous treatments as well as overall prognosis. The median survival in patients presenting with SVCS ranges from 1.5 to 9.5 months in the literature and must be kept in mind when tailoring an approach for these patients.[5] For patients with short life expectancy, the focus will be on short-term symptom relief. For patients with longer prognosis, more definitive treatment targeting not only the obstruction but the local tumors would provide better chances of control of SVCS.

REFERENCES

1. Armstrong BA, Perez CA, Simpson JR, et al. Role of irradiation in the management of superior vena cava syndrome. Int J Radiat Oncol Biol Phys 1987;13(4):531–9.
2. Markman M. Diagnosis and management of superior vena cava syndrome. Cleve Clin J Med 1999;66(1):59–61.
3. Ostler PJ, Clarke DP, Watkinson AF, et al. Superior vena cava obstruction: a modern management strategy. Clin Oncol (R Coll Radiol) 1997;9(2):83–9.
4. Perez-Soler R, McLaughlin P, Velasquez WS, et al. Clinical features and results of management of superior vena cava syndrome secondary to lymphoma. J Clin Oncol 1984;2(4):260–6.
5. Rowell NP, Gleeson FV. Steroids, radiotherapy, chemotherapy and stents for superior vena caval obstruction in carcinoma of the bronchus: a systematic review. Clin Oncol (R Coll Radiol) 2002;14(5):338–51.
6. Sculier JP, Evans WK, Feld R, et al. Superior vena caval obstruction syndrome in small cell lung cancer. Cancer 1986;57(4):847–51.
7. Chen YM, Yang S, Perng RP, et al. Superior vena cava syndrome revisited. Jpn J Clin Oncol 1995;25(2):32–6.
8. Spiro SG, Shah S, Harper PG, et al. Treatment of obstruction of the superior vena cava by combination chemotherapy with and without irradiation in small-cell carcinoma of the bronchus. Thorax 1983;38(7):501–5.
9. Presswala RG, Hiranandani NL. Pleural effusion and superior vena cava canal syndrome in Hodgkin's disease. J Indian Med Assoc 1965;45(9):502–3.
10. Lazzarino M, Orlandi E, Paulli M, et al. Primary mediastinal B-cell lymphoma with sclerosis: an aggressive tumor with distinctive clinical and pathologic features. J Clin Oncol 1993;11(12):2306–13.
11. Rice TW, Rodriguez RM, Light RW. The superior vena cava syndrome: clinical characteristics and evolving etiology. Medicine (Baltimore) 2006;85(1):37–42.
12. Parish JM, Marschke RF Jr, Dines DE, et al. Etiologic considerations in superior vena cava syndrome. Mayo Clin Proc 1981;56(7):407–13.
13. Schraufnagel DE, Hill R, Leech JA, et al. Superior vena caval obstruction. Is it a medical emergency? Am J Med 1981;70(6):1169–74.
14. Yellin A, Rosen A, Reichert N, et al. Superior vena cava syndrome. The myth–the facts. Am Rev Respir Dis 1990;141(5 Pt 1):1114–8.
15. Eren S, Karaman A, Okur A. The superior vena cava syndrome caused by malignant disease. Imaging with multi-detector row CT. Eur J Radiol 2006;59(1):93–103.
16. Stanford W, Jolles H, Ell S, et al. Superior vena cava obstruction: a venographic classification. AJR Am J Roentgenol 1987;148(2):259–62.
17. Kim HJ, Kim HS, Chung SH. CT diagnosis of superior vena cava syndrome: importance of collateral vessels. AJR Am J Roentgenol 1993;161(3):539–42.
18. Gauden SJ. Superior vena cava syndrome induced by bronchogenic carcinoma: is this an oncological emergency? Australas Radiol 1993;37(4):363–6.
19. Yu JB, Wilson LD, Detterbeck FC. Superior vena cava syndrome–a proposed classification system and algorithm for management. J Thorac Oncol 2008;3(8):811–4.
20. Schwartz EE, Goodman LR, Haskin ME. Role of CT scanning in the superior vena cava syndrome. Am J Clin Oncol 1986;9(1):71–8.
21. Bechtold RE, Wolfman NT, Karstaedt N, et al. Superior vena caval obstruction: detection using CT. Radiology 1985;157(2):485–7.
22. Conte FA, Orzel JA. Superior vena cava syndrome and bilateral subclavian vein thrombosis. CT and radionuclide venography correlation. Clin Nucl Med 1986; 11(10):698–700.

23. Podoloff DA, Kim EE. Evaluation of sensitivity and specificity of upper extremity radionuclide venography in cancer patients with indwelling central venous catheters. Clin Nucl Med 1992;17(6):457–62.

24. Hansen ME, Spritzer CE, Sostman HD. Assessing the patency of mediastinal and thoracic inlet veins: value of MR imaging. AJR Am J Roentgenol 1990;155(6): 1177–82.

25. Hartnell GG, Hughes LA, Finn JP, et al. Magnetic resonance angiography of the central chest veins. A new gold standard? Chest 1995;107(4):1053–7.

26. Loeffler JS, Leopold KA, Recht A, et al. Emergency prebiopsy radiation for mediastinal masses: impact on subsequent pathologic diagnosis and outcome. J Clin Oncol 1986;4(5):716–21.

27. Rice TW, Rodriquez RM, Barnette R, et al. Prevalence and characteristics of pleural effusions in superior vena cava syndrome. Respirology 2006;11(3):299–305.

28. Mineo TC, Ambrogi V, Nofroni I, et al. Mediastinoscopy in superior vena cava obstruction: analysis of 80 consecutive patients. Ann Thorac Surg 1999;68(1):223–6.

29. Porte H, Metois D, Finzi L, et al. Superior vena cava syndrome of malignant origin. Which surgical procedure for which diagnosis? Eur J Cardiothorac Surg 2000; 17(4):384–8.

30. Selcuk ZT, Firat P. The diagnostic yield of transbronchial needle aspiration in superior vena cava syndrome. Lung Cancer 2003;42(2):183–8.

31. Trinkle JK, Bryant LR, Malette WG, et al. Mediastinoscopy–diagnostic value compared to bronchoscopy: scalene biopsy and sputum cytology in 155 patients. Am Surg 1968;34(10):740–3.

32. Wilson LD, Detterbeck FC, Yahalom J. Clinical practice. Superior vena cava syndrome with malignant causes. N Engl J Med 2007;356(18):1862–9.

33. Jahangiri M, Taggart DP, Goldstraw P. Role of mediastinoscopy in superior vena cava obstruction. Cancer 1993;71(10):3006–8.

34. Callejas MA, Rami R, Catalan M, et al. Mediastinoscopy as an emergency diagnostic procedure in superior vena cava syndrome. Scand J Thorac Cardiovasc Surg 1991;25(2):137–9.

35. Herth F, Becker HD, Ernst A. Conventional vs endobronchial ultrasound-guided transbronchial needle aspiration: a randomized trial. Chest 2004;125(1):322–5.

36. Rowell NP, Gleeson FV. Steroids, radiotherapy, chemotherapy and stents for superior vena caval obstruction in carcinoma of the bronchus. Cochrane Database Syst Rev 2001;(4):CD001316.

37. Kaplan AP, Greaves MW. Angioedema. J Am Acad Dermatol 2005;53(3):373–88 quiz 389–92.

38. McDougall R, Sibley J, Haga M, et al. Outcome in patients with rheumatoid arthritis receiving prednisone compared to matched controls. J Rheumatol 1994;21(7):1207–13.

39. Wei L, MacDonald TM, Walker BR. Taking glucocorticoids by prescription is associated with subsequent cardiovascular disease. Ann Intern Med 2004;141(10): 764–70.

40. Adelstein DJ, Hines JD, Carter SG, et al. Thromboembolic events in patients with malignant superior vena cava syndrome and the role of anticoagulation. Cancer 1988;62(10):2258–62.

41. Ghosh BC, Cliffton EE. Malignant tumors with superior vena cava obstruction. N Y State J Med 1973;73(2):283–9.

42. Dombernowsky P, Hansen HH. Combination chemotherapy in the management of superior vena caval obstruction in small-cell anaplastic carcinoma of the lung. Acta Med Scand 1978;204(6):513–6.

43. Kane RC, Cohen MH. Superior vena caval obstruction due to small-cell anaplastic lung carcinoma. Response to chemotherapy. JAMA 1976;235(16): 1717–8.
44. Maddox AM, Valdivieso M, Lukeman J, et al. Superior vena cava obstruction in small cell bronchogenic carcinoma. Clinical parameters and survival. Cancer 1983;52(11):2165–72.
45. Tan EH, Ang PT. Resolution of superior vena cava obstruction in small cell lung cancer patients treated with chemotherapy. Ann Acad Med Singap 1995;24(6): 812–5.
46. Ahmann FR. A reassessment of the clinical implications of the superior vena caval syndrome. J Clin Oncol 1984;2(8):961–9.
47. Lonardi F, Gioga G, Graziella A, et al. Double-flash, large-fraction radiation therapy as palliative treatment of malignant superior vena cava syndrome in the elderly. Support Care Cancer 2002;10(2):156–60.
48. Pereira JR, Martins CJ, Ikari FK, et al. Neoadjuvant chemotherapy vs. radio-therapy alone for superior vena cava syndrome (SVCS) due to non-small cell lung cancer (NSCLC): preliminary results of a randomized phase II trial. Eur J Cancer 1999;35(Suppl 4):260.
49. Hennequin LM, Fade O, Fays JG, et al. Superior vena cava stent placement: results with the Wallstent endoprosthesis. Radiology 1995;196(2):353–61.
50. Irving JD, Dondelinger RF, Reidy JF, et al. Gianturco self-expanding stents: clin-ical experience in the vena cava and large veins. Cardiovasc Intervent Radiol 1992;15(5):328–33.
51. Rosch J, Uchida BT, Hall LD, et al. Gianturco-Rosch expandable Z-stents in the treatment of superior vena cava syndrome. Cardiovasc Intervent Radiol 1992; 15(5):319–27.
52. Bierdrager E, Lampmann LE, Lohle PN, et al. Endovascular stenting in neoplastic superior vena cava syndrome prior to chemotherapy or radiotherapy. Neth J Med 2005;63(1):20–3.
53. Greillier L, Barlesi F, Doddoli C, et al. Vascular stenting for palliation of superior vena cava obstruction in non-small-cell lung cancer patients: a future 'standard' procedure? Respiration 2004;71(2):178–83.
54. Kim YI, Kim KS, Ko YC, et al. Endovascular stenting as a first choice for the palli-ation of superior vena cava syndrome. J Korean Med Sci 2004;19(4):519–22.
55. de Gregorio Ariza MA, Gamboa P, Gimeno MJ, et al. Percutaneous treatment of superior vena cava syndrome using metallic stents. Eur Radiol 2003;13(4): 853–62.
56. Nagata T, Makutani S, Uchida H, et al. Follow-up results of 71 patients under-going metallic stent placement for the treatment of a malignant obstruction of the superior vena cava. Cardiovasc Intervent Radiol 2007;30(5):959–67.
57. Crowe MT, Davies CH, Gaines PA. Percutaneous management of superior vena cava occlusions. Cardiovasc Intervent Radiol 1995;18(6):367–72.
58. Oudkerk M, Kuijpers TJ, Schmitz PI, et al. Self-expanding metal stents for pallia-tive treatment of superior vena caval syndrome. Cardiovasc Intervent Radiol 1996;19(3):146–51.
59. Schindler N, Vogelzang RL. Superior vena cava syndrome. Experience with endo-vascular stents and surgical therapy. Surg Clin North Am 1999;79(3):683–94, xi.
60. Wilson P, Bezjak A, Asch M, et al. The difficulties of a randomized study in supe-rior vena caval obstruction. J Thorac Oncol 2007;2(6):514–9.

Electrolyte Complications of Malignancy

Robert F. Kacprowicz, MD[a,b,c,*], Jeremy D. Lloyd, MD[a,c]

KEYWORDS

- Malignancy • Electrolytes • Hypoglycemia • Hyponatremia
- Hypercalcemia • Hyperphosphatemia

Electrolyte abnormalities are perhaps the most common laboratory finding in patients with malignancies who present to the emergency department. Although most minor abnormalities have no specific treatment, severe clinical manifestations of several notable electrolytes occur with significant frequency in the setting of malignancy. If improperly treated, abnormalities of serum sodium, glucose, calcium, magnesium, and phosphorus may have serious consequences. A review of the most serious electrolyte abnormalities associated with malignancy follows.

HYPONATREMIA

Hyponatremia is a common electrolyte disorder, reported to occur in 3.8% of emergency department patients.[1] Among the population of emergency department patients with underlying malignancy, hyponatremia occurs most commonly with small cell lung cancers. Hyponatremia has been reported with other malignancies, including primary and metastatic malignancies of the brain, pancreatic adenocarcinoma, and prostate cancer.[2] Hyponatremia has also been reported in association with treatment with chemotherapeutic agents, particularly cisplatin and carboplatin.[3] Regardless of the associated malignancy, hyponatremia can present as either an incidental finding or with life-threatening severity. Correction of hyponatremia requires an understanding of both the rapidity with which the hyponatremia has developed as well as the potential complications of treatment.

[a] San Antonio Uniformed Services Health Education Consortium Residency in Emergency Medicine, San Antonio, TX, USA
[b] Department of Emergency Medicine, University of New Mexico School of Medicine, Albuquerque, NM, USA
[c] Department of Emergency Medicine, Wilford Hall USAF Medical Center, 2200 Bergquist Drive Suite 1/59 EMDS, Lackland AFB, TX 78236, USA
* Corresponding author. Department of Emergency Medicine, Wilford Hall USAF Medical Center, 2200 Bergquist Drive Suite 1/59 EMDS, Lackland AFB, TX 78236.
E-mail address: robert.kacprowicz@lackland.af.mil (R.F. Kacprowicz).

Emerg Med Clin N Am 27 (2009) 257–269
doi:10.1016/j.emc.2009.01.007
0733-8627/09/$ – see front matter. Published by Elsevier Inc.

emed.theclinics.com

Pathophysiology

Syndrome of inappropriate antidiuretic hormone

Hyponatremia associated with malignancy is most commonly caused by the syndrome of inappropriate antidiuretic hormone (SIADH) secretion. Ectopic secretion of arginine vasopressin (AVP) by tumor cells appears to play a significant role in the development of hyponatremia.[4] Small cell lung cancer is particularly notorious for elevated levels of circulating AVP despite serum hypotonicity.[4] Other hormones have been implicated in the pathogenesis of hyponatremia of malignancy, including atrial natriuretic peptide, but their ultimate contribution to hyponatremia remains somewhat unclear.[5]

Elevated levels of AVP in patients with malignancy cause hyponatremia primarily due to inappropriate retention of free water at the collecting-duct level despite relative serum hypotonicity.[6] Normally in the setting of hypotonicity, the secretion of AVP is suppressed. In malignancy, the release of AVP by tumor cells does not respond to changes in serum tonicity, and, as a result, AVP remains present in the circulation and results in cyclic AMP-mediated insertion of water channels in the collecting ducts (aquaporin 2).[7] The absorption of free water at the collecting-duct level results in worsening hypotonicity and inappropriately concentrated urine.[7] Clinically, the result is hyponatremia in an apparently euvolemic patient.

Renal salt wasting

Hyponatremia of malignancy has also been reported as a complication of chemotherapy. Both cisplatin and carboplatin have been reported to cause hyponatremia.[3] The mechanism for hyponatremia associated with chemotherapeutic drugs is believed to be renal salt wasting syndrome (RSWS). In this disease process, damage to the renal tubules with subsequent inability to retain sodium is thought to result in increased sodium loss.[8] Clinically, the patient will appear hyponatremic with euvolemia; however, the treatment of RSWS is sodium supplementation rather than water restriction. An elevated spot urine sodium level may suggest RSWS. In SIADH, urinary excretion of sodium is usually normal or decreased. Definitive diagnosis of RSWS, however, can only be made after measurement of daily sodium intake and excretion. RSWS is diagnosed when daily sodium intake is less than urinary excretion.[3] In extremis, however, treatment of hyponatremia due to RSWS is identical to the treatment of hyponatremia due to SIADH.

Clinical Manifestations

The clinical presentation of hyponatremia is largely related to the acuity with which the sodium has declined and has less direct correlation with the actual measured sodium. Levels of decline greater than 0.5 mEq/L/h appear to be more likely to result in serious sequelae, but considerable variation exists between individuals.[9] Most symptomatic individuals will have serum sodium less than 120 mEq/L; however, symptoms have been reported with sodium levels of 129 mEq/L or less.[7]

The brain appears to be the organ most sensitive to changes in the serum sodium level. If the rate of sodium decline outstrips the adaptive capabilities of the brain, symptoms of hyponatremia develop. When the rate of sodium decline is slower, the brain will adapt by expelling potassium and other osmotically active substances (osmolytes) to maintain normal cell volume. These osmolytes include amino acids, myoinositol, creatine, and creatine phosphate.[7] If, however, the rate of sodium decline exceeds the rate at which the brain can expel osmolytes, water shifts intracellularly down the osmotic gradient and results in cerebral edema.

In the setting of acute hyponatremia, the manifestations of the resultant cerebral edema may be severe and commonly include nausea, vomiting, headaches, seizures, coma, and respiratory arrest as the brain progressively swells. Increased intracranial pressure may eventually result in death due to herniation if hyponatremia is not treated.[10]

If hyponatremia develops more slowly, the symptoms may be less severe but present nonetheless. In the patient with chronic hyponatremia, brain cells have had more time to expel osmolytes and maintain near-normal cell volumes. Patients with chronic hyponatremia appear to be at very low risk of life-threatening cerebral edema and present with more subtle symptoms of brain dysfunction.[11] If the level of hyponatremia becomes severe (<120), seizures and altered mental status may still be present, and the sodium will require judicious correction.

In the emergency department, frequently, it will not be possible to determine the acuity of the hyponatremia. In the vast majority of out-of-hospital acquired cases of severe hyponatremia, the hyponatremia is chronic, and particular attention must be paid to the treatment of these patients, as they appear to be at much higher risk of treatment-related severe complications, particularly osmotic demyelination syndrome (ODS).[12] Rapidly correcting the sodium of a patient with chronic hyponatremia and minimal symptoms can be disastrous, so the decision to aggressively treat the hyponatremia should be made with a careful assessment of the risks and benefits of therapy.

OSMOTIC DEMYELINATION SYNDROME

The most feared complication of the treatment of hyponatremia is the ODS, previously known as central pontine myelinolysis. ODS was first reported in 1959 as a consequence of the treatment of a severely hyponatremic alcoholic patient.[13] Histologically, ODS is characterized by the destruction of oligodendrocytes and myelin in the central portion of the pons as well as the basal ganglia and cerebellum.[14] The clinical presentation of patients who develop ODS as a consequence of treatment of hyponatremia includes quadriparesis or quadriplegia, pseudobulbar palsy, and altered mental status. In the worst cases, patients develop the "locked-in syndrome," coma, and death days after treatment for hyponatremia.[15]

The pathophysiology of ODS is complex but appears to be related to brain cell shrinkage and concentrated ion damage during rapid changes in serum tonicity. As described previously, the response to chronic hyponatremia is the release of organic osmolytes from neurons. This adaptive response is protective in the setting of long-standing hyponatremia.[16] During acute correction, however, susceptible areas of the brain appear to be less able to reaccumulate these essential osmolytes.[17] In humans, areas less able to react to osmotic stress appear to be the neurons of the central pons, basal ganglia, and areas of the cerebellum, resulting in the potentially devastating constellation of neurologic findings seen in ODS.

ODS appears to be related to both the severity and the chronicity of hyponatremia. Chronic severe hyponatremia presents the greatest risk for development of ODS with rapid correction of the serum sodium. Most cases of ODS have been reported in patients with chronic hyponatremia of less than 120 mEq/L.[18] In the setting of malnutrition, however, ODS has been reported with higher serum sodium levels, a fact of significance in the treatment of hyponatremic cancer patients who are also at risk for malnutrition due to cachexia.[19]

The development of ODS also appears to be directly related to the rate of rise of the serum sodium. Rates greater than 12 mEq/L/24 h are strongly associated with the development of ODS.[11] Others have reported ODS occurring with rates of correction as low as 8 mEq/L/24 h, and the most recent consensus guidelines recommend limiting correction of the serum sodium to 8 mEq/L/24 h to avoid ODS.[6]

Treatment

Rapidly correcting the sodium of a patient with chronic hyponatremia and minimal symptoms can be disastrous, so the decision to aggressively treat the hyponatremia should be made with a careful assessment of the risks and benefits of therapy. In the emergency department, patients with altered mental status, seizures, respiratory depression, or coma require emergent correction of hyponatremia. If symptoms are milder, the risk of rapid correction of hyponatremia causing ODS generally outweighs the benefits, and these patients should be treated with simple fluid restriction.[6]

If the decision is made to correct hyponatremia emergently, the current treatment of choice is 3% saline infusion. Numerous formulas have been described for the calculation of free water excess, sodium deficit, and so on, but these formulas are cumbersome to use and not entirely reliable. A simpler approach is to infuse 1 cm^3/kg body weight of 3% NS per hour, which will result in an increase of 1 mEq/L serum sodium per hour.[6] Rates as high as 2 to 4 cm^3/kg/h can be tolerated in the short term when symptoms require, but in any case, treatment should be halted once one of three end points is reached:[1] resolution of symptoms,[2] serum sodium of 120 mEq/L is reached, or the daily limit of 8 mEq/L correction is reached.[6,12] Of course, hourly monitoring of the serum sodium is mandatory to prevent overcorrection.

In the event overcorrection does occur, relowering of the serum sodium through the infusion of D5W has the potential to reduce the risk of ODS and should be considered.[20]

If the patient experiences seizures, standard antiepileptic treatment should be used in addition to correction of the hyponatremia with hypertonic saline. Patients at risk for volume overload or with a history of congestive heart failure may be given 20 to 40 mg of furosemide to enhance diuresis.[6]

Disposition

Admission is warranted for any patient with significant symptoms due to hyponatremia. In the patient without symptoms, admission for fluid restriction and further evaluation is generally warranted if the serum sodium is at or less than 125 mEq/L, because symptoms most commonly develop below this level.[10] In the intermediate range (126–130 mEq/L), disposition should be based on the availability of expeditious follow-up care.

Future Directions

A new class of medications, arginine vasopressin receptor (AVPR) antagonists (vaptans), has recently been approved for clinical use and holds significant promise for future treatment of hyponatremia.[6] This is particularly true in cases of malignancy-associated SIADH, as the mechanism of action of these drugs would seem to be perfectly designed to counteract the effects of tumor-associated elevation of circulating AVP at the renal collecting-duct level. By interacting directly with the vasopressin receptor, AVPR antagonists cause an almost pure aquaresis by inhibiting the insertion of aquaporin 2 channels into the collecting duct and, thereby, result in a relative increase in serum sodium at the expense of free water diuresis.[21]

Several studies have demonstrated the usefulness of AVPR antagonists in euvolemic and hypervolemic hyponatremia.[22,23] The only AVPR antagonist currently approved for use is conivaptan, which has been approved for use in hospitalized patients with euvolemic hyponatremia due to SIADH, adrenal insufficiency, and hypo-thyroidism.[24] Conivaptan is given as an intravenous (IV) bolus of 20 mg over 30 minutes and then by continuous infusion of 20 to 40 mg over the next 24 hours.[24] Side effects due to conivaptan have reportedly been mild and most commonly include orthostatic dizziness, headache, and nausea.[23] Apart from a higher level of orthostatic dizziness in the treated patients, other side effects are comparable to those with placebo.[23]

The average increase in serum sodium in patients receiving vaptans in clinical trials has been 8 mEq/L, well within the safety range recommended for correction of hypo-natremia to prevent ODS.[25] Nine percent of patients had excessive rates of correction of sodium, but no cases of ODS have been reported thus far.[24]

No clinical trials have specifically addressed the use of vaptans for the treatment of severely symptomatic hyponatremia, either alone or as an adjunct to the use of hyper-tonic saline. Therefore, the use of vaptans in the emergency department, although enticing, cannot be currently recommended for the treatment of symptomatic hypona-tremia related to malignancy.

HYPOGLYCEMIA OF MALIGNANCY

Tumor-associated hypoglycemia is a relatively rare complication of malignancy. Hypoglycemia of malignancy has been described in association with 3 main etiologies. The most common cause is nonislet cell tumor hypoglycemia (NICTH).[26] Second, but perhaps more well known, is hypoglycemia due to insulin secretion by islet cell tumors of the pancreas.[27] Finally, end-stage metastatic carcinoma of nearly any source that has heavily infiltrated the liver or adrenal glands may cause hypoglycemia.[28] In the emergency department, the diagnosis and treatment of tumor-associated hypogly-cemia requires careful evaluation for other possible causes of hypoglycemia. When other causes have been excluded, treatment of tumor-associated hypoglycemia may be curative or palliative.

Pathophysiology

Perhaps the most well known cause of tumor-associated hypoglycemia is the insuli-noma of the pancreas. Insulinoma is a well-known but relatively rare tumor, occurring with an incidence of 1 to 4 per million people.[27] About 90% of insulinomas are benign, and surgical treatment is curative.[29] Insulinomas almost exclusively occur in the pancreas and represent deregulated production of insulin by beta cell tumors.[30]

In the case of NICTH, hypoglycemia is associated with a variety of tumors, including those of mesenchymal, epithelial, and hematopoietic origin.[29] The most common tumors among these tend to be fibrosarcomas, mesotheliomas, leiomyosarcomas, hepatomas, lung cancers, as well as gastric and pancreatic exocrine tumors.[29] NICTH appears to be caused by the secretion of insulin-like growth factor II, a circulating hormone normally synthesized in the liver, which is capable of activating insulin recep-tors and resulting in hypoglycemia.[31]

In the final instance, that of metastatic malignancy infiltrating the liver or adrenal glands, hypoglycemia is thought to occur either due to simple tissue destruction or due to as yet not fully identified secondary mechanisms, including secretion of tumor necrosis factor alpha, interleukins 1 and 6, or other mechanisms.[30] Research in animals tends to favor the latter explanation, as all of these compounds have been shown to cause profound hypoglycemia.[30]

Clinical Manifestations

Tumor-associated hypoglycemia presents no differently from hypoglycemia due to other mechanisms and should be suspected in any cancer patient with altered level of consciousness, obtundation, or bizarre behavior.[32]

Given the rarity of this disorder, however, a dedicated search for other causes of hypoglycemia should be undertaken before ascribing the symptoms and glucose level to tumor origin. If the patient is diabetic, effort must be taken to evaluate oral intake as well as medication regimen. A complete evaluation for infection or other organ dysfunction may also be warranted, because sepsis, renal failure, and liver failure are all well known, and more common, causes of hypoglycemia in the acutely ill emergency department patient.[29] In the absence of diabetes, infection, or organ dysfunction, evaluation for surreptitious use of insulin or other hypoglycemic agents should also be undertaken, because that is likely the most common cause of hypoglycemia in nondiabetics.[29]

When the patient is not known to have cancer, the diagnosis of tumor-associated hypoglycemia may be particularly difficult. Patients who are ultimately diagnosed with tumor-associated hypoglycemia have frequently suffered from long-standing bouts of recurrent fasting hypoglycemia without an identifiable cause. Admission for further evaluation of any patient with recurrent hypoglycemia with no identifiable cause is warranted, as evaluation of insulin, C-peptide and insulin-like growth factor I and II levels may be very helpful in elucidating the cause and expediting the further workup of suspected tumor-associated hypoglycemia.[26]

Treatment

Once hypoglycemia has been identified, the initial treatment is with glucose and glucose-containing solutions via standard regimens, followed by feeding once consciousness is normalized.

After the acute episode, treatment is directed at either curative or palliative measures. In the case of insulinomas and nonmetastatic tumors causing NICTH, surgical excision may be curative.[30] If operative treatment is not possible due to coexisting disease, invasive disease, and/or metastatic disease, treatment in concert with an endocrinologist may provide relief from symptomatic hypoglycemia. Depending on the tumor, regimens composed of prednisone with or without somatostatin analogs appear to be effective in eliminating the occurrence of symptomatic hypoglycemia.[26]

Disposition

As discussed above, admission is warranted for any patient with hypoglycemia that is recurrent or for which no readily reversible cause can be found (eg, diabetic who has skipped a meal). This is particularly true of those in whom a diagnosis of tumor-associated hypoglycemia has not been made as expedited workup and surgical treatment may be curative.

In the case of a patient with known insulinoma, NICTH, or metastatic malignancy, the ultimate disposition decision should be made in concert with the patient, the patient's oncologist, and likely in consultation with an endocrinologist.

HYPERCALCEMIA

Hypercalcemia is the most common serious electrolyte abnormality in adults with malignancies. It has been reported to occur in 20% to 40% of patients during their disease.[33] The presence of hypercalcemia associated with cancer is associated with a poor prognosis, as this metabolic disorder may result in numerous life-threatening complications, including severe dehydration, bradycardia, seizures, pancreatitis, and coma. Up to 50% of patients die within 30 days of detection of elevated calcium levels.[34]

Pathophysiology

Hypercalcemia typically complicates cancers of the breast, lung, head, and neck as well as leukemia and multiple myeloma. There appears to be a complex set of interactions between bone synthesis and degradation that is responsible for the elevated calcium. Contrary to expectations, bone metastasis does not seem to be required. In patients with hypercalcemia and squamous cell carcinoma of the lung, only 16% have bone lesions, whereas patients with numerous bony metastases from small cell carcinoma of the lung rarely have hypercalcemia.[35]

Four mechanisms have been described to be responsible for hypercalcemia associated with malignancy. Local osteolytic hypercalcemia, comprising 20% of cases, results from significant increase in osteoclastic bone resorption in areas surrounding malignant cells within marrow space. The most common type of hypercalcemia associated with cancer is referred to as humoral hypercalcemia of malignancy (HHM), responsible for 80% of the cases. It is primarily caused by the secretion of humoral factors from tumor cells. Parathyroid hormone-related peptide is the major humoral factor responsible for the elevated serum calcium. This peptide increases bone resorption and decreases renal calcium excretion. Hodgkin's disease, non-Hodgkin's lymphoma, myeloma, and some solid tumors secrete the active form of Vitamin D, 1,25-dihydroxyvitamin D (1,25(OH)2D), causing hypercalcemia due to enhanced intestinal absorption of calcium and increased osteoclastic bone resorption. Finally, there are rare reports of hypercalcemia due to ectopic secretion of PTH by tumors such as ovarian carcinoma.[36,37]

Calcium exists in the extracellular state in a free ionized form or bound to other molecules. The typical laboratory value for total calcium ranges from 8.5 to 10.5 mg/dL. Only about 45% of the total calcium is biologically active in the ionized form. Therefore, laboratory measurement of total calcium can be misleading, since the serum albumin level significantly influences it. Mathematical formulas correcting for albumin have proven to be inaccurate.[38] Since many patients with advanced malignancy will be hypoalbuminemic, an ionized calcium level should be measured if available.

Clinical Manifestations

Hypercalcemia of malignancy typically presents with nonspecific signs and symptoms. The emergency physician must consider calcium abnormalities in any cancer patient with mental status changes or lethargy. In general, calcium levels do not correlate with symptoms, since the acuity of the rise is more important. Hypercalcemia associated with cancer normally occurs rapidly and, therefore, the symptoms of hypercalcemia are more dramatic. The patients suffer from severe dehydration, nausea, vomiting, confusion, and stupor. Patients with more chronic hypercalcemia will complain of anorexia, nausea, vomiting, constipation, polydipsia, polyuria, and memory loss.[39]

Gastrointestinal symptoms, such as nausea, vomiting, anorexia, and constipation, result from smooth muscle relaxation. Neurologically patients may be lethargic, hypotonic, confused, or comatose. The elevated calcium can cause polyuria, nephrolithiasis, and dehydration. The dehydration can exacerbate the hypercalcemia by renal efforts to expand volume through proximal tubule resorption of sodium and calcium. The calcium can also directly affect the electric conduction pathways of the heart.

Electrocardiogram features include shortened heart-rate corrected QT intervals, broadened T waves, and first-degree atrioventricular block.

Since hypercalcemia presents in advanced tumors, the malignancy will be evident on presentation, and as mentioned earlier, prognosis is poor. Breast carcinoma and multiple myeloma are the exceptions, as they may typically be successfully treated in the hypercalcemic patient. Successful urgent treatment of the elevated calcium allows time to treat the underlying malignancy and may ultimately result in long-term survival for the patient.

Treatment

Efforts to rapidly lower serum calcium levels in the severely hypercalcemic patient should be made alongside efforts to reverse complications and identify the underlying cause. The most common cause for hypercalcemia in the ED, primary hyperparathyroidism, can be confirmed by elevated PTH level. In contrast, hypercalcemia associated with malignancy will have a low to normal PTH level except for the rare cases due to ectopic production of PTH. Overall management of the hypercalcemic patient should be considered in the context of the underlying disease and clinical condition. Treatment should focus on improving quality of life, mental status, and kidney function and allow for effective therapy. The physician should also note that in certain situations, such as when no improvement in quality of life can be expected and pain control is difficult, the effects of hypercalcemia might provide relief in the dying patient with advanced metastatic disease.

Basic strategies for lowering calcium levels in mild cases focus on decreasing calcium intake and increasing mobility of the patient. Calcium should be removed from parenteral feedings and any oral supplementation stopped. Any other medications that may lead to high calcium levels, such as lithium, vitamin D, thiazides, or calcitriol should also be discontinued. A consideration of reduction in sedatives and analgesics, which may lead to increased weight-bearing mobility, will also be beneficial.

More aggressive therapy is required for successful treatment of severe hypercalcemia (>14 mg/dL) (**Table 1**). Patients are typically profoundly dehydrated; therefore, initial treatment should begin with volume expansion. Recommendations call for IV hydration with normal saline at 200 to 500 mL/h. Volume expansion increases calcium

Table 1		
Treatment for severe hypercalcemia		
Therapy	**Dosing**	**Frequency**
Rehydration	200–500 mL/h of 0.9% NaCl	Qd x 1–5 d
Furosemide	20–40 mg IV (after hydration)	Q12–24 h
Pamidronate	60–90 mg IV over 2–4 h	Once
Zoledronate	4 mg IV over 15–30 min	Once
Calcitonin	4–8 IU/kg SC	Q12–24 h
Gallium nitrate	200 mg/m^2 IV over 24 h	Qd x 5 d
Glucocorticoids	200–300 mg hydrocortisone IV	Qd x 5 d
Dialysis	—	—

Data from Bringhurst FR, Demay MB, Kronenberg HM. Hormones and disorders of mineral metabolism. In: Kronenberg HM, Melmed S, Polonsky KS, et al, editors. Williams textbook of endocrinology. 11th edition. Philadelphia: Saunders; 2008.

excretion by decreasing passive reabsorption in the proximal tubule and the loop of Henle. Once dehydration is corrected and adequate urine output is achieved, a loop diuretic can be added to further augment urinary calcium excretion. Thiazide diuretics decrease urinary calcium excretion and should be avoided. Fluid status and electrolytes require strict monitoring to prevent overcorrection or fluid overload.[36]

Bisphosphonates have become the mainstay of treatment for hypercalcemia. They bind to bone hydroxyapatite and inhibit osteoclast formation and function, leading to decreased bone resorption. The most commonly used bisphosphonates in the United States, zoledronate and pamidronate, may be administered IV and are generally well tolerated. Studies of pamidronate report decreases in calcium levels in 24 hours, with normalization of calcium in 90% of patients in 3 to 4 days. These effects usually last for 3 to 4 weeks.[40] Pamidronate is much less expensive per dose; however, zoledronate has the advantage of ease of administration (see **Table 1**).

With the widespread use of bisphosphonates, the emergency physician should be aware of their potential toxicities. Up to one-third of patients report acute phase reactions usually within 2 days of treatment. The acute phase reactions, typically bone pain and flu-like symptoms, will resolve within 1 to 2 days. Patients are also at risk for hypophosphatemia, hypermagnesemia, and hypocalcemia. Close monitoring of electrolytes will allow for appropriate supplementation or treatment as indicated. The more feared complication of IV bisphosphonates is nephrotoxicity occurring in 6% to 10% of patients.[41] Patients with moderate renal insufficiency (glomerular filtration rate >30 mL/min) may still receive full dosing; however, it may be prudent to prolong the rate of delivery to 2 to 3 times the normal time of infusion. For more severe renal insufficiency, patient should forego bisphosphonates and instead undergo dialysis with low-calcium dialysate.[42] Recent literature also associates osteonecrosis of the jaw with bisphosphonate use. At particular risk are those patients with breast cancer or multiple myeloma with an incidence as high as 10%.[43] Ophthalmologic complications, such as anterior uveitis, scleritis, and conjunctivitis can also occur after administration.[41]

Other second-line agents may be of help when bisphosphonates fail or contraindications prevent their use. Salmon calcitonin increases renal excretion of calcium and decreased osteoclast-mediated bone resorption. Calcitonin has the most rapid reduction in calcium levels, with full results in 12 to 24 hours. However, the total reduction serum calcium is quite small and transient. Calcitonin has been shown to be more effective when combined with glucocorticoids. Steroids lower calcium levels by inhibiting the effects of vitamin D. They are particularly suited for treatment associated with lymphomas and elevated 1,25(OH)2 vitamin D. Steroids have a slow onset of action, and effects are not seen for 4 to 10 days.[36,44] Historically, plicamycin (mithramycin) was used to treat hypercalcemia before the wide availability of bisphosphonates. Although reported to be effective in up to 80% of patients, its use was limited by side effects that include renal insufficiency, hepatotoxicity, thrombocytopenia, and coagulopathy.[35] The manufacturer discontinued production in 2000 due to decreased demand. Gallium nitrate is also very effective in lowering calcium levels through potent inhibition of bone resorption. However, treatment requires a continuous infusion over 5 days and side effects, including pleural effusions, pulmonary infiltrates, optic neuritis, and nephrotoxicity, complicate its effectiveness.[45]

Occasionally, certain patients with severe hypercalcemia of malignancy may be poor candidates for standard therapy with IV fluids and bisphosphonates. In this situation, dialysis may be indicated. This would typically be reserved for patients with renal insufficiency or heart failure. The standard hemodialysis fluid must be modified to be virtually calcium-free. Other modifications to the dialysis fluid can be considered on an individual basis based on the particular electrolyte abnormalities of the patients. For example, enrichment of the dialysate with phosphorus proved to result in rapid correction of all metabolic abnormalities after the patient had failed other medical therapy.

Disposition

Patients with severe hypercalcemia associated with malignancy will require close monitoring as treatment is begun to reduce calcium levels as well as diagnose and treat the underlying illness. An intensive-care setting may be required as the patient is initially rehydrated to watch for signs of electrolyte abnormalities with cardiac monitoring and frequent laboratory testing. These patients will need strict measurement of fluid input and output to determine overall hydration status. Ongoing care should be guided by response to treatment and overall underlying disease.

Future Directions

Although the majority of patients with hypercalcemia will respond to saline hydration and treatment with bisphosphonates, as many as one-quarter with HHM will fail to achieve normocalcemia. The resistance to treatment is attributed to renal calcium reabsorption and inadequate inhibition of bone resorption. New treatments are in development that target the molecular pathway leading to osteoclast recruitment and differentiation. This is known as the receptor activator of nuclear factor-kB (RANKL) ligand system. Monoclonal antibodies directed against RANKL and recombinant osteoprotegerin (OPG) are novel agents that interfere with this system. Animal studies comparing OPG to bisphosphonate to treat hypercalcemia of malignancy have been promising. Morony and colleagues reported rapid reversal of hypercalcemia with OPG, which occurred faster and lasted longer than treatments with bisphosphonates. Hypercalcemia eventually returned despite clear evidence of significantly suppressed bone resorption but to a lesser extent than those treated with bisphosphonates.[46] A small study in 2007 has also shown cinacalcet (calcimimetic) to be effective in lowering calcium levels in patients with elevated PTH related to parathyroid carcinoma. The patients had advance disease and had failed standard treatment with IV bisphosphonates and surgery. Two-thirds of the patients achieved a reduction in their serum calcium level of at least 1 mg/dL.[47]

These agents will require further testing to determine their overall safety and effectiveness in treating hypercalcemia of malignancy. It remains to be determined if they can be produced in a more cost effective manner as well as with better outcomes than those of standard treatment with bisphosphonates.

HYPOMAGNESEMIA

Hypomagnesemia frequently complicates the stay of hospitalized patients and seems to correlate with severity of illness. Up to 60% of patients in intensive care have low serum magnesium. Symptoms become present at levels below 1.2 mg/dL; however, they may be very nonspecific and are often overlooked. Most often, the symptoms manifest as neurologic or cardiovascular abnormalities. A neurologic examination may reveal muscle weakness, tremors, hyperreflexia, or tetany. Other neurologic abnormalities range from dizziness, apathy, and irritability to seizures and coma. Magnesium-deficient patients are also at risk for multiple dysrhythmias, ranging from atrial fibrillation, multifocal atrial tachycardia, and supraventricular tachycardia to premature ventricular contractions, ventricular tachycardia, or even ventricular fibrillation. Patients with congestive heart failure, who are treated with diuretics or digoxin, are particularly prone to dysrhythmias.[48]

Patients with any serious signs or symptoms of hypomagnesemia should be treated with IV magnesium. The standard dosage is 2 to 4 g of 50% magnesium sulfate diluted in saline or dextrose over 1 hour. Faster administration may result in bradycardia, heart block, or hypotension. These symptoms may be exacerbated with pre-existing renal insufficiency or atrioventricular block.

HYPOPHOSPHATEMIA

Hypophosphatemia is an additional electrolyte abnormality common to hospitalized patients. It is also a known complication of bisphosphonate treatment. Mild to moderate hypophosphatemia is usually asymptomatic; however, if the serum phosphate levels drop below 1.0 mg/dL, serious clinical symptoms may be present. The symptoms are related to impaired energy metabolism from decreased ATP production. As a result, all organ systems can be affected. Clinical signs and symptoms range from muscle weakness, rhabdomyolysis, impaired cardiac contractility, respiratory depression, confusion, seizures, and coma.

Although mild to moderate hypophosphatemia can be corrected with oral phosphate supplementation, severe symptomatic hypophosphatemia should be corrected with IV phosphate. Two standard formulations, potassium phosphate or sodium phosphate, are available for use in various suggested regimens. Weight-based regimens recommend 2.5 to 5 mg/kg over 6 hours.[49] More aggressive treatment with up to 30 mmol potassium phosphate IV in 50 mL saline over 2 h has also proven to be safe.[50] The faster replacement therapy takes place, the more likely that side effects will occur. Side effects of IV phosphate repletion include hypocalcemia, hyperkalemia, volume overload, hypernatremia, metabolic acidosis, and hyperphosphatemia.[51]

SUMMARY

A thorough working knowledge of the diagnosis and treatment of life-threatening electrolyte abnormalities in cancer patients, especially hyponatremia, hypoglycemia, and hypercalcemia, is essential to the successful practice of emergency medicine. Newer therapies that are targeted at the pathophysiological mechanisms underlying these electrolyte abnormalities have recently been developed and appear to have a promising future.

REFERENCES

1. Lee CT, Guo HR, Chen JB. Hyponatremia in the emergency department. Am J Emerg Med 2000;18:264–8.
2. Sverha JJ, Borenstein M. Emergency complications of malignancy. In: Tintinalli J, Kelen GD, Stapcyzinski JS, editors. Emergency medicine: a comprehensive study guide. 5th edition. New York: McGraw-Hill; 2000. p. 1408–14.
3. Cao L, Prashant J, Sumoza D. Renal salt wasting in a patient with cisplatin-induced hyponatremia. Am J Clin Oncol 2002;25:344–6.
4. Sorensen JB, Andersen MK, Hansen HH. Syndrome of inappropriate secretion of antidiuretic hormone (SIADH) in malignant disease. J Intern Med 1995;238: 97–110.
5. Johnson BE, Chute JP, Rushin J, et al. A prospective study of patients with lung cancer and hyponatremia of malignancy. Am J Respir Crit Care Med 1997;156: 1669–78.
6. Verbalis JG, Goldsmith SR, Greenberg A, et al. Hyponatremia treatment guidelines 2007: expert panel recommendations. Am J Med 2007;120:S1–21.

7. Yeong-Hau LH, Shapiro JI. Hyponatremia: clinical diagnosis and management. Am J Med 2007;120:653–8.
8. Vassal G, Rubie C, Kalifa C, et al. Hyponatremia and renal sodium wasting in patients receiving cisplatinum. Pediatr Hematol Oncol 1987;4:337–44.
9. Arieff A, Llach F, Massey SG. Neurological manifestations and morbidity of hyponatremia: correlation with brain water and electrolytes. Medicine 1976;55:121–9.
10. Lauriat SM, Berl T. The hyponatremic patient: practical focus on therapy. J Am Soc Nephrol 1997;8:1599–607.
11. Sterns RH. Severe symptomatic hyponatremia: treatment and outcome. A study of 64 cases. Ann Intern Med 1987;107:656–64.
12. Decaux G, Soupart A. Treatment of symptomatic hyponatremia. Am J Med Sci 2003;326(1):25–30.
13. Adams RD, Victor M, Mancall ED. Central pontine myelinolysis: a hitherto undescribed disease occurring in alcoholic and malnourished patients. AMA Arch Neurol Psychiatry 1959;81(2):154–72.
14. Wright DG, Laureno R, Victor M. Pontine and extrapontine myelinolysis. Brain 1979;102:361–5.
15. Rabinstein AA, Wijdicks EF. Hyponatremia in critically ill neurological patients. Neurologist 2003;9(6):290–300.
16. Yancey PH, Clark ME, Hand SC, et al. Living with water stress: evolution of osmolyte systems. Science 1982;217:1214–22.
17. Lien YH. Role of organic osmolytes in myelinolysis. A topographic study in rats after rapid correction of hyponatremia. J Clin Invest 1995;95:1579–86.
18. Soupart A, Decaux G. Therapeutic recommendations for management of severe hyponatremia: current concepts on pathogenesis and prevention of neurologic complications. Clin Nephrol 1996;46:149–69.
19. Laureno R. Central pontine myelinolysis following rapid correction of hyponatremia. Ann Neurol 1983;13:232–42.
20. Soupart A, Ngassa M, Decaux G. Therapeutic relowering of the serum sodium in a patient after excessive correction of hyponatremia. Clin Nephrol 1999;51:383–6.
21. Knepper MA. Molecular physiology of urinary concentrating mechanism: regulation of aquaporin water channels by vasopressin. Am J Phys 1997;272:F3–12.
22. Verbalis JG, Bisaha JG, Smith N. Novel vasopressin V1A and V2 antagonist (conivaptan) increases serum sodium concentration and effective water clearance in patients with hyponatremia. J Card Fail 2004;10(Suppl 4):S27.
23. Ghali JK, Koren MJ, Taylor JR, et al. Efficacy and safety of oral conivaptan: a V1A/V2 vasopressin receptor antagonist, assessed in a randomized, placebo-controlled trial in patients with euvolemic or hypervolemic hyponatremia. J Clin Endocrinol Metab 2006;91(6):2145–52.
24. Vaprisol (package insert). Deerfield (IL): Astellas Pharma US; 2005.
25. Oh M. Management of hyponatremia and clinical use of vasopressin antagonists. Am J Med Sci 2007;332:101–5.
26. Nayar MK, Lombard MG, Furlong NJ, et al. Diagnosis and management of non-islet cell tumor hypoglycemia. Endocrinologist 2006;16(4):227–30.
27. Service FJ. Hypoglycemic disorders. N Engl J Med 1995;91:505–10.
28. de Groot JW, Rikhof B, van Doorn J, et al. Non-islet cell tumour induced hypoglycaemia: a review of the literature including two new cases. Endocr Relat Cancer 2007;14:979–93.
29. Le Roith D. Tumor-induced hypoglycemia. N Engl J Med 1999;341:757–8.
30. Marks V, Teale JD. Tumours producing hypoglycaemia. Endocr Relat Cancer 1998;5:111–29.

31. Daughaday WH, Trivedi B. Measurement of derivatives of proinsulin-like growth factor-II in serum by radioimmunoassay directed against the E-domain in normal subjects and patients with nonislet cell tumor hypoglycemia. J Clin Endocrinol Metab 1992;75:110–5.

32. Strewler GJ. Humoral manifestations of malignancy. In: Kronenberg HM, Shlomo M, Polonsky KS, et al, editors. Williams textbook of endocrinology. 11th edition. Philadelphia: Saunders; 2008. p. 1803–17.

33. Mundy GR, Guise TA. Hypercalcemia of malignancy. Am J Med 1997;103:134–45.

34. Ralston SH, Gallagher SJ, Patel U, et al. Cancer associated hypercalcemia: morbidity and mortality: clinical experience in 126 treated patients. Ann Intern Med 1990;112:499–504.

35. Barri YM, Knochei JP. Hypercalcemia and electrolyte disturbances in malignancy. Hematol Oncol Clin North Am 1996;10:775–80.

36. Stewart AF. Clinical practice. Hypercalcemia associated with cancer. N Engl J Med 2005;352(4):373–9.

37. Nussbaum SR, Gaz RD, Arnold A. Hypercalcemia and ectopic secretion of parathyroid hormone by an ovarian carcinoma with rearrangement of the gene for parathyroid hormone. N Engl J Med 1990;323:1324–8.

38. Ladenson JH, Lewis JW, McDonald JM, et al. Relationship of free and total calcium in hypercalcemic conditions. J Clin Endocrinol Metab 1978;48:393–7.

39. Shepard MM, Smith JW. Hypercalcemia. Am J Med Sci 2007;334(5):381–5.

40. Body JJ. Current and future directions in medical therapy: hypercalcemia. Cancer 2000;88:3054–8.

41. Layman R, Olson K, Van Poznak C. Bisphosphonates for breast cancer. Hematol Oncol Clin North Am 2007;21(2):341–67.

42. Koo WS, Jeon DS, Ahn SJ, et al. Calcium-free hemodialysis for the management of hypercalcemia. Nephron 1996;72:424–8.

43. Woo SB, Hellstein JW, Kalmar JR. Systematic review: bisphosphonates and osteonecrosis of the jaws. Ann Intern Med 2006;144(10):753–61.

44. Ariyan CE, Sosa JA. Assessment and management of patients with abnormal calcium. Crit Care Med 2004;32:S146–54.

45. Kinirons MT. Newer agents for the treatment of malignant hypercalcemia. Am J Med Sci 1993;305:403–6.

46. Morony S, Warmington K, Adamu S, et al. The inhibition of RANKL causes greater suppression of bone resorption and hypercalcemia compared with bisphosphonates in two models of humoral hypercalcemia of malignancy. Endocrinology 2005;146:3235–43.

47. Shoback D. Cinacalcet hydrochloride reduces hypercalcemia in patients with parathyroid carcinoma. Nat Clin Pract Endocrinol Metab 2007;3(12):794.

48. Gibbs MA, Tayal VS. Electrolyte disturbances. In: Marx JA, Hockberger RS, Walls RM, et al, editors. Rosen's emergency medicine: concepts and clinical practice. 6th edition. Philadelphia: Saunders; 2006. p. 1933–53.

49. Taylor BE, Huey WY, Buchman TG, et al. Treatment of hypophosphatemia using a protocol based on patient weight and serum phosphorus level in a surgical intensive care unit. J Am Coll Surg 2004;198(2):198–204.

50. Charron T, Bernard F, Skrobik Y. Intravenous phosphate in the intensive care unit: more aggressive repletion regimens for moderate and severe hypophosphatemia. Intensive Care Med 2003;29(8):1273–8.

51. Gaasbeek A. Hypophosphatemia: an update on its etiology and treatment. Am J Med 2005;118(10):1094–101.

Adrenal Insufficiency and Other Adrenal Oncologic Emergencies

Yael R. Taub, MD[a,b], Robert W. Wolford, MD, MMM[a,b,*]

KEYWORDS

- Adrenal insufficiency • Corticosteroids
- Aldosterone • Megestrol • Pheochromocytoma
- Hypothalamic-pituitary axis • Incidentaloma

The adrenal gland, and its endocrine function, is frequently affected by a variety of malignancies involving other organs or by their treatment. In addition, primary adrenal cancers can alter normal adrenal function and response to stress. The failure to recognize chronic or acute adrenal insufficiency or epinephrine excess can cause significant morbidity or mortality.

ADRENAL GLAND OVERVIEW

The adrenal glands are paired organs, weighing between 3 and 5 g, located at the superior poles of the kidneys, and they are well visualized by computed tomography (CT) and magnetic resonance imaging (MRI). Aldosterone, cortisol, and epinephrine are the 3 major products of the gland. Additionally, the adrenal gland is responsible for the production of small amounts of estrogen, androgen, and 2 androgen precursors. The cortex of the adrenal gland is composed of 3 layers: glomerulosa, fasciculata, and the reticularis. The glomerulosa, composing ~ 5% of the mature cortex, is responsible for aldosterone production, which has a key role in the maintenance of salt balance and blood pressure regulation. Cortisol is secreted by the fasciculata, which makes up about 70% of the cortex. Sex hormones and their precursors are products of the reticularis. Epinephrine and norepinephrine are produced by chromaffin cells located in the central zone of the gland, the medulla. Important oncologic-related adrenal disorders to be identified in the emergency department (ED) include the following: (1) inadequate cortisol production (adrenal insufficiency), (2) excess cortisol production, and (3) excess catecholamine release (pheochromocytoma).

[a] Department of Emergency Medicine, University Hospitals Case Medical Center, 11100 Euclid Avenue, Bolwell 3700, Cleveland, OH 44106, USA
[b] Department of Emergency Medicine, Case Western Reserve University School of Medicine, Cleveland, OH 44106, USA
* Corresponding author. Department of Emergency Medicine, University Hospitals Case Medical Center, 11100 Euclid Avenue, Bolwell 3700, Cleveland, OH 44106.
E-mail address: robert.wolford@UHhospitals.org (R. W. Wolford).

Emerg Med Clin N Am 27 (2009) 271–282
doi:10.1016/j.emc.2009.01.008
0733-8627/09/$ – see front matter © 2009 Elsevier Inc. All rights reserved.
emed.theclinics.com

Regulation of Cortisol Production, the Hypothalamic-Pituitary-Adrenal Axis

Cortisol production is closely regulated by positive and negative feedback loops involving the hypothalamus, anterior pituitary, and the adrenal gland (**Fig. 1**). A number of different stressors stimulate the hypothalamus to secrete the corticotrophin-releasing hormone (CRH), which reaches the anterior pituitary via the hypophyseal portal vasculature. In response to CRH, the anterior pituitary secretes adrenocortico-tropic hormone (ACTH). ACTH stimulates cells in the fasciculata layer of the adrenal cortex, which, in turn, secrete cortisol. Cortisol is essential in the body's response to stress, impacting immune function, vascular tone, as well as lipid, protein, and carbohydrate metabolism. Via a negative feedback loop, cortisol inhibits the secretion of CRH and ACTH. Knowledge of the hypothalamic-pituitary-adrenal (HPA) axis is essential in understanding how cancer, or its treatment, may produce inadequate or excess levels of cortisol and cause the resulting syndromes.

Regulation of the Renin-Angiotensin-Aldosterone System

The production of aldosterone is frequently impaired by processes causing primary adrenal insufficiency, and hypoaldosteronism contributes to a number of the clinical findings that are observed. The regulation of aldosterone production is summarized in **Fig. 2**. Briefly, juxtaglomerular cells associated with the afferent arterioles of glomer-ular afferent arterioles are the primary site of renin secretion. In response to inade-quate vascular volume, renin is secreted. Renin in turn converts angiotensinogen to angiotensin I, which is then converted to angiotensin II (primarily in the lungs). Angio-tensin II has numerous biologic effects, one of which is the stimulation of the adrenal cortex glomerulosa layer to synthesize and secrete aldosterone. Aldosterone acts on the thick ascending loop of Henle to increase sodium reabsorption, leading to volume expansion. Decreased levels of sodium and chloride are sensed by the macula densa cells of the distal tubule (associated with inadequate vascular volume) and also stim-ulate renin release. Elevated sodium and chloride levels (associated with adequate vascular volume) lead to inhibition of renin secretion.

From this discussion, it is clear that in primary adrenal insufficiency, processes leading to hypoadrenalism will be associated with salt wasting and inadequate intra-vascular volume. The findings of dehydration, hypotension, hyponatremia, and

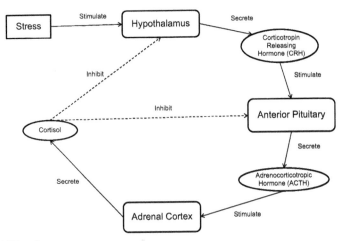

Fig. 1. The HPA axis.

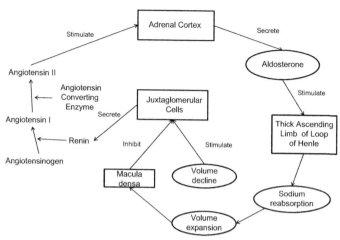

Fig. 2. Renin-angiotensin-aldosterone system.

hyperkalemia may occur. In addition, primary adrenal masses with unregulated aldosterone production will lead to hypertension and hypokalemic alkalosis (Conn's syndrome).

ADRENAL INSUFFICIENCY SYNDROMES (HYPOCORTISOLISM)

Adrenal insufficiency is a syndrome caused by inadequate amounts of cortisol caused by a variety of primary adrenal diseases and by processes affecting the HPA axis. It may be classified as either primary (diseases affecting the adrenal gland itself) or as secondary (inadequate ACTH production) leading to inadequate cortisol production. The differentiation between primary and secondary adrenal insufficiency may be suggested by an examination of the skin and serum sodium and potassium levels (**Table 1**). Oncologic-associated causes of adrenal insufficiency are listed in **Table 2**.

Presenting Signs and Symptoms of Adrenal Insufficiency

Nonspecific symptoms are typical of adrenal insufficiency and include fatigue, anorexia, abdominal complaints (nausea, vomiting, and pain), dehydration, and orthostatic hypotension. Although hyperpigmentation (particularly noticeable in non–sunlight-exposed areas) is characteristic of primary adrenal insufficiency, it is not usually present in patients with secondary adrenal insufficiency. Laboratory findings that may be present include hyponatremia, hyperkalemia, and hypoglycemia (particularly in the fasting state). However, these are found less frequently in secondary adrenal insufficiency. Anemia, lymphocytosis, and eosinophilia may be present as well. Although mild presentations are the norm, acute adrenal crisis has life-threatening

Table 1		
Primary versus secondary adrenal insufficiency		
Characteristics	**Primary**	**Secondary**
Skin	Hyperpigmented (especially in non–sun-exposed areas)	Pale (not due to anemia)
Sodium levels	Low	Low or normal
Potassium levels	High	Normal

Table 2
Oncologic-associated causes of adrenal insufficiency

Primary Adrenal Insufficiency	Secondary Adrenal Insufficiency
Bilateral adrenal metastasis	Pituitary or hypothalamus surgery
Bilateral adrenal hemorrhage	Pituitary or hypothalamus tumors
Bilateral adrenalectomy	Pituitary hemorrhage (apoplexy)
—	Pituitary or brain irradiation
—	Discontinuation of chronic glucocorticoid therapy
—	Medications (eg, megestrol acetate)

presentations. This is particularly true in patients with underlying malignancies, in whom there is a greater risk of decompensation due to an inability to appropriately respond to any stress with cortisol production. In primary adrenal insufficiency, the signs and symptoms of hypocortisolism are also affected by the degree to which aldosterone production is reduced. Most cases of adrenal crisis occur in patients with known underlying adrenal insufficiency. In addition to the signs and symptoms discussed here, another important presentation is that of hypotension, which responds poorly to aggressive fluid resuscitation and vasopressors. Abdominal pain, weakness, loss of consciousness, and fever often confuse the diagnosis of adrenal crisis, delaying appropriate management.

Management of Adrenal Insufficiency

Key to the management of adrenal insufficiency is its early recognition, which requires a high index of suspicion. As discussed above, the symptoms and signs of adrenal insufficiency can be vague and delay its diagnosis. In both primary and secondary adrenal insufficiency, treatment centers on the replacement of cortisol, and in the case of primary adrenal insufficiency, also mineralocorticoids (**Table 3**).[1] Patients presenting with acute adrenal crisis will require admission, generally to an intensive care unit. The disposition of patients with suspected chronic adrenal insufficiency will be dependent on their presentation and underlying illnesses.

Testing for Adrenal Insufficiency

In a state of stress, a random cortisol level should be sufficient to indicate if the patient has a decreased ability to respond with increased glucocorticoid production. The level of appropriate response has been debated, although 20 μg/dL is typically accepted as the cutoff point. If the patient has a cortisol level greater than 20 μg/dL, adrenal function is generally adequate, and if it is less than 4 μg/dL, it indicates that it is deficient.[4] Ranges, though, have been cited from 10 to 34 μg/dL.[5] Morning cortisol levels are not particularly applicable in the ED setting.

The insulin tolerance test (ITT) is the gold standard for testing the HPA axis. Unfortunately, in very sick patients, inducing hypoglycemia is not always reasonable, as this in itself can induce an acute adrenal crisis. In the ITT, insulin is used to induce hypoglycemia, following which cortisol levels are then measured, as hypoglycemia is a potent stimulus of the HPA axis. A cortisol level greater than 18 to 25 μg/dL is generally considered to represent an adequate response.[4–6] Blood sugar levels are usually reduced to less than 40 mg/dL, which makes the ITT impractical in the very ill, the elderly, and patients with a history of cardiac disease, seizures, or cerebrovascular disease.[6] In addition, some patients may have an appropriate cortisol response to hypoglycemia and still have underlying adrenal insufficiency.

Table 3 Management of adrenal insufficiency	
Acute Adrenal Insufficiency (Crisis)	**Chronic Adrenal Insufficiency**
Pretreatment laboratory tests Electrolytes, calcium, glucose baseline cortisol, ACTH, renin, & aldosterone	Confirmed by diagnostic testing
ACTH stimulation test with cortisol level 30 min postinjection	—
Fluid resuscitation (D5 NS or NS)	—
Glucocorticoid administration Hydrocortisone 100–200 mg IV, repeat 50–100 mg IV every 6 h until confirmatory tests available Dexamethasone 6–10 mg IV (use if ACTH stimulation test is to be performed, does not interfere with cortisol-level measurement)	Glucocorticoid administration: Hydrocortisone 15–25 mg daily po or Cortisone acetate 25–37.5 mg daily po divided bid or tid Mineralocorticoid replacement (only in primary adrenal insufficiency): Fludrocortisone 0.05–0.2 mg po daily
—	Hydrocortisone "stress" dosing Minor: 30–50 mg daily Major: initially 150 mg in D5 W over 24 h & then 100 mg in next 24 h followed by taper
Admit to ICU	—

Data from Refs. [1-3].

The metyrapone test is an overnight HPA axis test that works by blocking the negative feedback inhibition of cortisol. Metyrapone inhibits the adrenal enzyme 11-hydroxylase, prevents the conversion of 11-deoxycortisol to cortisol, and causes a drop in serum cortisol. The induced drop in cortisol in a patient with an intact HPA axis should cause the pituitary to release ACTH, which stimulates the adrenal glands to increase cortisol production (demonstrated by a rise in 11-deoxycortisol).[7] It is used infrequently as it can also precipitate an acute adrenal crisis. In addition, other drugs may affect metyrapone's clearance, leading to errors in interpretation. The metyrapone test, however, is a useful reference test to assess other methods for determining adrenal insufficiency, such as the ACTH stimulation testing.[8]

ACTH (Cosyntropin) stimulation testing is currently the preferred test for adrenal insufficiency. Two separate doses have been validated in the literature, with uncertainty as to which is more effective.[5,6,9] This test assesses only the ability of the adrenal cortex to respond with increased cortisol production and not of the HPA axis as a whole. In this test, either 1 μg (low dose–physiologic) or 250 μg (standard–supraphysiologic) of cosyntropin, a synthetic derivative of ACTH that acts directly on the adrenal cortex, is administered after a baseline cortisol level is drawn. A repeat cortisol level is drawn 30 minutes later. Independent of the cosyntropin dose used, either of the following 2 results is considered evidence of an appropriate adrenal response: (1) a cortisol level of 20 to 25 μg/dL or (2) an increase of more than 9 μg/dL above the baseline value. It has been suggested that only the peak cortisol level be used and not the change in cortisol as a basis for treatment.[10] An abnormal ACTH stimulation test effectively "rules in" adrenal insufficiency, however a normal test does not completely "rule it out," as the reported range of sensitivities of the test are 65% to 100%.[11]

In summary, for suspected adrenal insufficiency, it is reasonable to obtain a random cortisol level and consider an ACTH stimulation test in the ED. However, therapy for adrenal insufficiency should not be delayed to wait for test results. Dexamethasone can also be used in the ED, since it does not interfere with the results of the ACTH stimulation test.

Cancer as a Cause of Adrenal Insufficiency

Although rare, patients with cancer of nearly any type can present with adrenal insufficiency. To cause adrenal insufficiency, 90% of the adrenal gland must be nonfunctional before adrenal function is detectably impaired.[12] Often this is through metastasis. The most common cancers to metastasize to the adrenals are lung, breast, and melanoma. Renal, thyroid, and colon cancer have also been known to metastasize to the adrenals. These metastases may be either unilateral or bilateral, although the larger bilateral tumors tend to be the symptomatic ones. Patients with hypoadrenalism often present with the same nonspecific symptoms frequently associated with the cancer itself, including fatigue, weakness, and weight loss. Nonspecific abdominal pain is present in 50% of these patients. A high index of suspicion must be maintained to appropriately evaluate for adrenal insufficiency in these patients and to initiate treatment in a timely fashion.

In addition to a site of metastasis, the adrenal glands can also be a primary site of cancer as well, causing acute adrenal insufficiency once the tumor has reached a critical mass. Adrenal masses are found in at least 3% of people older than 50; years at autopsy. Nearly all are nonfunctional, and 1 in 4,000 is malignant.[13] The size of the tumor correlates with its likelihood of being a primary adrenal adenocarcinoma. One-quarter of tumors larger than 6 cm are malignant, whereas only 2% of those less than 4 cm are malignant.[13] Patients with tumors 6 cm or larger in size tend to have poor outcomes. With regard to adrenal function, tumors larger than 3 cm tend to be hyperfunctioning, whereas smaller tumors are likely to be nonfunctional.

Tumors of the adrenal cortex may also be benign or malignant, and both may or may not be functional. The tumors that cause virilization through excess sex steroid production tend to be malignant adrenocortical carcinomas, whereas the cortisol- and aldosterone-secreting tumors tend to be benign. Those that are functional result in hypercortisolism or hyperaldosteronism. These tumors are evaluated radiologically and by assessing the appropriate hormone levels. If less than 12 cm, laparoscopic adrenalectomy is the treatment of choice for benign tumors. Complete surgical resection is the treatment of choice for stage I to III adrenocortical carcinomas. Adjuvant therapies, such as chemotherapy and radiation, may then be employed.[11]

Cancer Treatments and Their Effects on the HPA Axis

Apart from the havoc that cancer or its adrenal metastases might wreak on a patient, treatment for cancer can cause an unending series of complications by affecting the function of the HPA axis and the adrenal glands. Commonly, cancer patients have difficulties with oral intake secondary to decreased appetite. Megestrol acetate, a synthetic progesterone-like compound, is commonly used as an appetite stimulant in these patients. It has been noted that the extended use of megestrol can cause Cushing-like symptoms, and its rapid withdrawal can precipitate acute adrenal insufficiency. Although the exact mechanism of action is unclear, megestrol appears to suppress the HPA axis through its glucocorticoid-like activity. It is incumbent, therefore, to keep the HPA axis in mind when patients currently taking megestrol, or having recently withdrawn from megestrol, present with symptoms such as fatigue, weight loss, and electrolyte disturbances.[14] The duration of megestrol use does not appear to be particularly relevant, as cortisol levels in healthy volunteers were noted to be suppressed after a single low dose.[15] On the other hand, patients treated with high-dose megestrol are likely to have Cushing-like features, such as moon facies, striae, myopathy, and centripetal obesity. New-onset diabetes has been seen as well. Agonist effects are more likely to occur in those on longer courses with higher doses of megestrol.[16] Symptoms of adrenal insufficiency may become clinically apparent when (1) a patient misses a dose of megestrol, leading to sudden withdrawal of gluco-corticoid activity; (2) a patient experiences significant stressors (eg, infection); (3) the megestrol binds the glucocorticoid receptors, preventing more effective endogenous glucocorticoids; and (4) greater inhibition of the HPA axis compared with its ability to signal peripheral metabolic effects of glucocorticoids.[16] Cancer patients may require stress dosing of steroids while on megestrol and should be counseled not to stop this medication on their own.[17]

Other common medications, such as opioids, can also induce adrenal insufficiency. A case report[18] published in 2005 describes a patient whose HPA axis was sup-pressed by chronic transdermal fentanyl use. In addition, morphine has also been shown in rats to increase the levels of corticosteroid-binding globulin and thereby reducing active free corticosteroid blood levels. This may lead to immune compro-mise, as glucocorticoids are needed to maintain normal immune function.[19]

There is a large literature describing the affects of the treatment of brain cancer and brain metastasis on the HPA axis. Studies have shown neuroendocrine dysfunction years after treatment from primary brain tumors to be more common than initially postulated.[20] Symptoms may start subtly but can have a major effect on the quality of life.[20] Now that survival rates for adults with primary brain tumors are higher than those in patients in the past, there is a notable increase in neuroendocrine dysfunction in these patients, even years after treatment. The source of the dysfunction is likely at the level of the hypothalamus as opposed to the pituitary gland, since the former is more sensitive to radiation. Up to 21% of patients with nonpituitary primary brain tumors treated with irradiation will develop secondary glucocorticoid deficiency.[21] The likelihood of developing dysfunction is dependent on the duration and intensity of the brain irradiation. At lower radiation doses, ACTH suppression is practically unheard of, especially if the primary malignancy was not a pituitary or nasopharyngeal cancer.[22] Irradiation for acute lymphoblastic leukemia also places a patient at risk for subsequent neuroendocrine dysfunction.

One of the most commonly used medications in patients with cancer that affect endogenous glucocorticoid production is supplemental steroids. Steroids are often added to patients' regimens for a variety of reasons, including pain control, reduction of edema in patients with CNS malignancies, prevention of vomiting, and prevention of common allergic reactions associated with chemotherapies. They are also used as a component of treatment regiments for patients with prostate cancer, breast cancer, thymomas, as well as some hematologic malignancies. In contrast, glucocorticoids used as monotherapy or adjuvant therapy in patients with lung cancer actually decrease survival.[23] In patients with multiple myeloma, dexamethasone may induce remission in up to 40% of patients with baseline good prognostic indicators and is quite useful for patients who would be unable to tolerate more toxic marrow-suppres-sive agents. Steroids are also used as maintenance therapy in multiple myeloma patients.[24] Side effects, unfortunately, are particularly common in the elderly. Adverse effects include hyperglycemia, bacterial and fungal infections, reactivation of herpes, psychosis, hypertension, and fluid retention.

Regardless of their intended use, administration of glucocorticoids in various formu-lations can cause Cushing-like effects and subsequent adrenal insufficiency if the steroid need is no longer met, with either reduction of dose, withdrawal, or increased stress on the patient. Adrenal atrophy may be caused by the negative feedback inhibition of cortisol secretion in patients receiving long-term glucocorticoid therapies.[1] Again, these patients may present to the ED with vague effects related to their underlying cancer or therapy-related complaints. The ED physician must consider adrenal insufficiency when evaluating these patients. Depending on the severity and type of the insufficiency, typical laboratory abnormalities may or may not be present.

Finally, there are particular medications that can affect cortisol levels in any sick patient in the ED. One of the most common is etomidate, an induction agent often used for rapid sequence intubation. Etomidate lowers cortisol levels and responsiveness to ACTH by inhibiting 11-beta-hydroxylase. Patients taking spironolactone, ketoconazole, and estrogens may also have lower cortisol levels or decreased responsiveness to cortisol induction by ACTH or its equivalent.[25]

CORTISOL EXCESS

Although rarely is the diagnosis definitively made nor treatment initiated in the ED, it is important to consider cortisol excess in the appropriate clinical settings and to refer the patient for further evaluation. Patients with untreated cortisol excess have a much increased morbidity and mortality, which can be reduced by appropriate management.

The most common cause of hypercortisolism (Cushing's syndrome) in the United States is the use of exogenous glucocorticoids. If exogenous glucocorticoids as an etiology is eliminated, the remaining mechanisms (**Table 4**) may be classified as ACTH dependent (cortisol secreted in response to excess ACTH) or independent (cortisol secreted independent of ACTH stimulation).[26,27] The most common oncologic-associated cause (70% of all nonpharmacologic cases) is ACTH secretion by a pituitary adenoma (Cushing's disease).[26,27] The majority of remaining cases are evenly split between ACTH-secreting nonpituitary tumors (frequently lung) and cortisol-producing primary adrenal tumors.[26,27]

Excessive cortisol causes a myriad of signs and symptoms, the most classic of which include central obesity, moon facies, deep purple striae, supraclavicular fat pad, and proximal muscle weakness. Other features are summarized in **Box 1**. It is rare, however, for patients to have all of the classic findings, and in many instances the signs and symptoms overlap with a host of other medical conditions (eg, depression, obesity, alcoholism).[27] A not uncommon ED presentation of patients with Cushing's syndrome is that of psychiatric illness, most often depression.[28] The diagnosis of Cushing's syndrome/disease is a difficult one to make on clinical grounds. In addition,

Table 4 Nonpharmacologic causes of Cushing's syndrome	
ACTH Independent	**ACTH Dependent**

Adrenal tumors (15%)
  Adrenal adenoma
  Adenocarcinoma
	ACTH-producing pituitary tumor (70%)

Other (rare)
  Pigmented nodular
    adrenocortical disease
  Massive macronodular
    adrenocortical disease
	ACTH-producing nonpituitary tumor (15%)

Data from Refs. [26,27].

Box 1
Symptoms and signs of hypercortisolism

Central obesity

Striae

Facial rounding (moon faces)

Supraclavicular fat pads

Hypertension

Hirsutism

Oligomenorrhea

Erectile dysfunction

Plethora

Muscle weakness (typically proximal)

Osteoporosis

Psychiatric illness (especially depression)

Lethargy

Acne

Bruising

Poor wound healing

Alopecia

Hyperkalemia

Glucose intolerance/diabetes mellitus

---

laboratory testing to confirm the diagnosis is infrequently available in a timely fashion in the ED. Fortunately, rarely does Cushing's syndrome require emergent management. It is important for the diagnosis to be considered in the ED differential diagnosis of illnesses with overlapping signs and symptoms and for this group of patients to be referred for further testing in a timely manner.

CATECHOLAMINE EXCESS
Pheochromocytoma

Adrenal tumors may also involve the medulla, and these tend to be neuroendocrine tumors. The most known of these are pheochromocytomas, which are catecholamine-producing tumors derived from chromaffin cells. They typically present in the fourth or fifth decade of life and are typically solitary and unilateral.[29] Only about 10% of pheochromocytomas are malignant.[29] Unfortunately, the malignant potential is often not determined until the pheochromocytoma has already metastasized. Sites of metastasis include lungs, liver, lymph nodes, and bone, the latter of which bodes the best prognosis. Malignant tumors are usually larger, extra-adrenal, and associated with higher levels of catecholamines in the plasma or urine. The presence of the succinate dehydrogenase family of gene mutations is also more likely in malignant tumors.[30] Symptoms associated with pheochromocytomas are the direct result of elevated catecholamine levels. Typically, both norepinephrine and epinephrine are released with a predominance of norepinephrine; however, any combination of catecholamine release may be seen, with some tumors also producing dopamine.[31] The classic symptom triad of episodic headache, diaphoresis, and palpitations or tachycardia or 1 or more of the components of the triad have been reported in 90% of patients in some series.[29] In other series, 50% of patients may have sustained hypertension, and 10% to 15% may have orthostatic hypotension.[29] Additional symptoms may include anxiety, chest pain, weakness, and weight loss. ED management focuses on the timely referral of patients with suspicious signs and symptoms. If management of the hypertension is necessary in the ED, an alpha-blocking agent (typically phentolamine) should be initiated before the use of any beta-blocking agent, to prevent the severe hypertension associated with unopposed alpha-receptor stimulation. In addition, the ED physician should avoid medications that may cause catecholamine release (eg, opiates, histamine, sympathomimetics) or that block catecholamine reuptake (eg, tricyclic antidepressants).[29]

No treatment has proven consistently successful in the treatment of pheochromocytomas. Surgical resection may be curative in some instances. Debulking surgery is often used for symptomatic relief, and radiation therapy, for bony metastases. Chemotherapy may be used after surgery, but complete remission is unfortunately rare (5%).[11]

MANAGEMENT OF INCIDENTALOMAS

With ongoing improvements in imaging (particularly CT and MRI) and their ever increasing ED use, the discovery of "incidental" adrenal masses (unexpectedly found on a radiograph examination for a nonadrenal indication) and decisions about their further evaluation are common problems. Autopsy studies of patients older than 50 years of age show an incidence of adrenal masses of at least 3%. The incidence of adrenal masses (1 cm or greater) found on radiographic imaging is comparable with an incidence of about 4%. The likelihood of finding an incidentaloma increases with age. Incidentalomas are present in less than 1% of patients younger than 30 years and in approximately 7% of individuals older than 70 years.[32] The etiology of the mass varies from benign to life threatening and is summarized in **Box 2**. The majority of adrenal masses are non–hypersecreting benign adenomas (~70%).[13,32,33] In patients with known nonadrenal cancers, nearly 75% will be metastases compared with less than 1% without known malignancies.[13] As the size of the mass increases, so does the likelihood that it is malignant. In addition, benign lesions that are hypersecreting cortisol, aldosterone, catecholamines, or sex hormones can cause substantial

---

Box 2
Etiology of adrenal incidentalomas

Adrenocortical adenoma

Adrenocortical carcinoma

Pheochromocytoma

Metastasis

Other adrenal tumors

Hematoma

Cysts

Infection

Other

morbidity and mortality. As a result, all patients with newly discovered adrenal masses in the ED should be referred for further radiographic and biochemical evaluation.[13] The main questions to be answered are (1) is the mass hypersecreting and (2) is the mass malignant?

SUMMARY

Normal function of the adrenal gland can be disrupted not only by metastases of non-adrenal cancers but also by their treatment. In addition, tumors of the adrenal gland itself can cause disease by hypersecretion of a variety of hormones, adrenal gland destruction with inadequate production of cortisol, and by metastasis to other sites. Although rare, abnormal adrenal function, especially adrenal insufficiency, should be considered in appropriate clinical settings, as failure to recognize and treat can result in significant morbidity and mortality. Adrenal "incidentaloma" is a frequent finding of abdominal radiologic studies. All patients with an unexpected adrenal mass should be referred for further evaluation.

REFERENCES

1. Hafner S, Allolia B. Management of adrenal insufficiency in different clinical settings. Expert Opin Pharmacother 2005;6(14):2407–17.
2. Salvatori R. Adrenal insufficiency. JAMA 2005;294:2481–8.
3. Boulillon R. Acute adrenal insufficiency. Endocrinol Metab Clin North Am 2006;35: 767–75.
4. Toogood A, Stewart P. Hypopituitarism: clinical features, diagnosis, and management. Endocrinol Metab Clin North Am 2008;37:235–61.
5. Sakharova O, Inzucchi S. Endocrine assessments during critical illness. Crit Care Clin 2007;23:467–90.
6. Reimondo G, Bovio S, Allasino B, et al. Secondary hypoadrenalism. Pituitary 2008;11:147–54.
7. Endert E, Ouwehand A, Fliers E, et al. Establishment of reference values for endocrine tests. Part IV: adrenal insufficiency. Neth J Med 2005;63(11):435–43.
8. Annane D, Maxime V, Ibrahim F, et al. Diagnosis of adrenal insufficiency in severe sepsis and septic shock. Am J Respir Crit Care Med 2006;174:1319–26.
9. Kazlauskaite R, Evans A, Villabona C, et al. Corticotropin tests for hypothalamic-pituitary adrenal insufficiency: a meta-analysis. Published ahead of print as. J Clin Endocrinol Metab 2008;10.1210/jc.2008-0710.
10. Dickstein G, Saiegh L. Low-dose and high-dose adrenocorticotropin testing: indications and shortcomings. Curr Opin Endocrinol Diabetes Obes 2008;15(3): 244–9.
11. Kuruba R, Gallagher S. Current management of adrenal tumors. Curr Opin Oncol 2008;20:34–46.
12. Sirachainan E, Kalemkerian G. Unusual presentations of lung cancer: case 2. Adrenal insufficiency as the initial manifestation of non-small-cell lung cancer. J Clin Oncol 2002;20(23):4598–600.
13. NIH State-of-the-Science Statement on management of the clinically inapparent adrenal mass ("incidentaloma"). NIH Consens State Sci Statements 2002;19(2): 1–23.
14. Raedler T, Jahn H, Goedeken B, et al. Acute effects of megestrol on the hypothalamic-pituitary-adrenal axis. Cancer Chemother Pharmacol 2003;52:482–6.
15. Briggs MH, Briggs M. Glucocorticoid properties of progestogens. Steroids 1973; 22:555–9.

16. Mann M, Koller E, Murgo A, et al. Glucocorticoidlike activity of megestrol. A summary of Food and Drug Administration experience and review of the literature. Arch Intern Med 1997;157:1651–6.

17. Meacham L, Mazewski C, Krawiecki N. Mechanism of transient adrenal insufficiency with megestrol acetate treatment of cachexia in children with cancer. J Pediatr Hematol Oncol 2003;25(5):414–7.

18. Oltmanns KM, Fehm HL, Peters A. Chronic fentanyl application induces adrenocortical insufficiency. J Intern Med 2005;257:478–80.

19. Noch B, Wich M, Cicero T. Chronic exposure to morphine increases corticosteroid-binding globulin. J Pharmacol Exp Ther 1997;282(3):1262–8.

20. Arlt W, Hove U, Muller B, et al. Frequent and frequently overlooked: treatment-induced endocrine dysfunction in adult long-term survivors of primary brain tumors. Neurology 1997;49(2):498–506.

21. Agha A, Sherlock M, Brennan S, et al. Hypothalamic-pituitary dysfunction after irradiation of nonpituitary brain tumors in adults. J Clin Endocrinol Metab 2005; 90(12):6355–60.

22. Darzy K, Shalet S. Absence of adrenocorticotropin (ACTH) neurosecretory dysfunction but increased cortisol concentration and production rates in ACTH-replete adult cancer survivors after cranial irradiation for nonpituitary brain tumors. J Clin Endocrinol Metab 2005;90(9):5217–25.

23. Keith B. Systematic review of the clinical effect of glucocorticoids in nonhematologic malignancy. BMC Cancer 2008;8:84.

24. Ludwig H, Strasser-Weipple K, Schreder M, et al. Advances in the treatment of hematological malignancies: current treatment approaches in multiple myeloma. Ann Oncol 2007;18(Suppl 9):ix64–70.

25. Arafah B. Review: hypothalamic pituitary adrenal function during critical illness: limitations of current assessment methods. J Clin Endocrinol Metab 2006; 91(10):3725–45.

26. Loriaux DL. The adrenal. In: Dale DC, editor. ACP Medicine Online. WebMD, Inc. October 2004 Update, Endocrinology:Chapter IV.

27. Nieman LK, Ilias I. Evaluation and treatment of Cushing's syndrome. Am J Med 2005;118:1340–6.

28. Preuss JM. Adrenal emergencies. Top Emerg Med 2001;23(4):1–13.

29. Fung MM, Viveros OH, O'Connor DT. Diseases of the adrenal medulla. Acta Physiol (Oxf) 2008;192:325–35.

30. Eisenhofer G, Borstein S, Brouwers F, et al. Malignant pheochromocytoma: current status and initiatives for future progress. Endocr Relat Cancer 2004;11: 423–36.

31. Reisch N, Peczkowska M, Janusezewicz A, et al. Pheochromocytoma: presentation, diagnosis, and treatment. J Hypertens 2006;24:2331–9.

32. Young WF. The incidentally discovered adrenal mass. N Engl J Med 2007;356: 601–10.

33. Cicala MV, Sartorato P, Mantero F. Incidentally discovered masses in hypertensive patients. Best Pract Res Clin Endocrinol Metab 2006;20(3):451–66.

Renal Complications in Oncologic Patients

Melissa L. Givens, MD, MPH[a,b],*, Joy Wethern, DO, FACEP, FACMT[a]

KEYWORDS

- Acute renal failure • Tumor lysis syndrome
- Thrombotic microangiopathy • Nephrotoxicity • Malignancy

Acute renal failure (ARF) can be one of the many complications associated with malignancy and, unfortunately, often harbors a worse prognosis for the afflicted patient. Insult to the kidneys can occur for a variety of reasons in the oncologic patient. The kidneys are susceptible to injury from malignant infiltration, damage by metabolites of malignant cells, nephrotoxic drugs including chemotherapeutic agents, tumor lysis syndrome (TLS), radiation, septicemia associated with immune suppression, cast nephropathy, complications of bone marrow transplant (BMT), and autoimmune phenomena. This article focuses on several of these etiologies, such as TLS and thrombotic microangiopathy (TMA), which are unique threats faced by the oncologic patient. Therapeutic and diagnostic drug-induced nephrotoxicity, although common in all disease states, is also briefly reviewed. Nephrotoxic complications of chemotherapeutic agents warrant a separate discussion and are reviewed elsewhere in this issue.

EPIDEMIOLOGY

It is difficult to quantify the extent of renal complications associated with malignancy, as renal dysfunction can be present before the identification of malignancy, coincide with the diagnosis of malignancy, or be a secondary or tertiary effect of treatment. Several studies have examined the occurrence of renal failure in patients with specific malignancies, such as leukemia, lymphoma, and multiple myeloma. About 20% to 40% of newly diagnosed multiple myeloma patients have evidence of renal impairment.[1,2] Renal failure in lymphoma and leukemia is also well described. The incidence of renal complications in leukemia patients undergoing chemotherapy has been reported to be 30% or greater.[3,4] Patients undergoing BMT for leukemia have a 50% risk of renal complications.[4] Unfortunately, the presence of ARF is also an

[a] Department of Emergency Medicine, Carl R. Darnall Army Medical Center, 36000 Darnall Loop, Fort Hood, TX 76544, USA
[b] Department of Military and Emergency Medicine, Uniformed Services University of the Health Sciences, 4301 Jones Bridge Road, Bethesda, MD, USA
* Corresponding author. Department of Emergency Medicine, Carl R. Darnall Army Medical Center, 36000 Darnall Loop, Fort Hood, TX 76544.
E-mail address: melissa.givens@us.army.mil (M.L. Givens).

Emerg Med Clin N Am 27 (2009) 283–291
doi:10.1016/j.emc.2009.01.001
0733-8627/09/$ – see front matter. Published by Elsevier Inc.
emed.theclinics.com

independent risk factor for a poor prognosis.[5–8] A reasonable approach to these patients in the emergency department (ED) is to consider prerenal, renal, and postrenal etiologies, since more than 1 type of azotemia may be present (listed in **Table 1**).[9]

PRERENAL AZOTEMIA

Prerenal azotemia is commonly encountered in cancer patients and can be due to multiple mechanisms, including poor oral intake, early satiety, vomiting, and diarrhea. Elderly cancer patients are particularly prone to dehydration, which should be corrected promptly to minimize further renal injury.

RENAL AZOTEMIA
Malignant Infiltration

Malignant infiltration of the kidneys is very common in leukemia and lymphoma. Fortunately, the presence of malignancy-related infiltration does not always coincide with renal dysfunction, and severe infiltration is rare.[10,11] Leukemic or lymphoma infiltration of the kidneys can present with a variety of signs and symptoms, varying from mild proteinuria to florid ARF. The only way to diagnose infiltration is by renal biopsy; thus, in the emergent evaluation of malignancy-associated renal failure, it is important to exclude more easily identifiable causes for the dysfunction.[10,11] Once identified, infiltration of the kidney is addressed by aggressively treating the primary malignancy with chemotherapy.

Tumor Lysis Syndrome

TLS is a metabolic emergency secondary to the breakdown of a large tumor burden with release of intracellular contents into the extracellular space and systemic circulation. Factors that contribute to TLS are the type of malignancy, its responsiveness to chemotherapy, rapidity of cell turnover, and tumor burden. It is clinically defined by the triad of hyperuricemia, hyperphosphatemia, and hyperkalemia, whereas elevated serum lactate dehydrogenase (LDH) levels, hypocalcemia, and ARF are secondary findings. Although the potassium and phosphate are primarily derived from

Table 1
Causes of acute renal failure in cancer patients

Prerenal Failure	Renal (Intrinsic) Failure	Postrenal Failure
Volume loss	Acute tubular necrosis	Intrarenal obstruction
Poor intake	Shock	Urate crystals
Diarrhea	Nephrotoxic compounds	Light chain (myeloma)
Vomiting	Intravascular hemolysis	Extrarenal obstruction
Sepsis	Acute interstitial nephritis	Retroperitoneal
Drugs	Cancer infiltration	fibrosis
NSAIDs	Postinfectious	Ureteral/bladder
ACE inhibitors	glomerulonephritis	outlet obstruction
Sinusoidal obstruction syndrome	Allergic nephritis	
(hepatorenal syndrome)	Vascular nephritis	
Capillary leak syndrome (IL-2)	Thrombotic	
	microangiopathy	
	Renal vasculature	
	thrombosis or stenosis	
	Glomerulonephritis	

Abbreviations: ACE, angiotensin-converting enzyme; IL-2, interleukin-2.

cytoplasmic contents, the uric acid is a product of nucleic acid breakdown. Hypocalcemia is secondary to calcium downregulation in the setting of hyperphosphatemia. TLS can occur spontaneously, but it is more commonly seen following the initiation of chemotherapy. Cancers such as acute lymphocytic leukemia (ALL), acute myelogenous leukemia (AML), Burkitt's lymphoma, and large solid tumors are more prone to TLS after the initiation of chemotherapy. Spontaneous TLS has been described in AML and ALL and is usually associated with marked hyperuricemia in the absence of hyperphosphatemia. It is thought that in spontaneous TLS, the released phosphorus is reutilized by new cancer cells.

TLS usually appears within 1 to 5 days of a chemotherapy session. Symptoms are nonspecific and include nausea, vomiting, fatigue, and weakness. Altered mental status, cardiac dysrhythmias, autonomic instability, and ARF are common findings on presentation. A recent study by Montesinos and colleagues[12] evaluated predisposing factors in an attempt to develop a predictive model for TLS in patients with AML. In this study of 772 adults, 130 (17%) developed TLS. Multivariate analysis showed that pretreatment LDH levels above laboratory normal values, creatinine (Cr) >1.4 mg/dL, uric acid >7.5 mg/dL, and white blood cell counts >25 × 10(9)/L were independent risk factors for TLS. Prechemotherapy laboratory evaluation should be performed to assess the risk for development of TLS and to assist in the decision to initiate prophylactic therapy in high-risk patients.

The goal of therapy and prophylaxis (**Table 2**) is to promote excretion of metabolic products, to prevent renal failure, and decrease uric acid production. The mainstay of therapy to date has been hydration or hyperhydration. Two to 4 times maintenance hydration with normal saline or isotonic sodium bicarbonate solutions to assist with urine alkalinization is generally recommended. Urine alkalinization with sodium bicarbonate to a goal pH between 7.0 and 8.0 may prevent precipitation of uric acid in the renal tubules; however, there are no experimental studies confirming any benefit to urine alkalinization. One study that compared urine alkalinization to hydration alone showed hydration to be just as effective in minimizing uric acid precipitation.[13] Furthermore, alkalinization may encourage deposition of calcium phosphate in organs of patients with existing hyperphosphatemia. Current recommendations are to alkalinize urine with a bicarbonate solution only in patients with existing metabolic acidosis. Alkalinization should continue until uric acid ceases to climb and is closer to a normal reference range of 2.0 to 8.0; however, reference ranges differ for males, females, and pediatric versus adult populations. If bicarbonate alkalinization fails to achieve a urine pH greater than 7.0, intravenous (IV) acetazolamide may be given to well-hydrated patients to decrease bicarbonate reabsorption in the proximal renal tubules.[14] Bicarbonate therapy should be discontinued once uric acid levels normalize, if serum bicarbonate is greater than 30 mEq/L, or if urine pH is more than 8.0. It is also important to simultaneously manage other symptomatic electrolyte abnormalities, such as hyperkalemia and hypocalcemia.

Allopurinol, rasburicase, and dialysis for renal failure are also appropriate adjunctive therapies to hydration. Allopurinol works by inhibiting xanthine oxidase, which prevents further production of uric acid but does nothing to decrease existing pools. Allopurinol also leads to increased levels of hypoxanthine and xanthine in the urine. Even when combined with hydration, allopurinol may fail to prevent renal compromise in up to 25% of cases.[15] Concurrent urine alkalinization with the use of allopurinol has been standard, but is now somewhat controversial. Rasburicase is a newer and highly effective alternative to allopurinol, which does not require simultaneous urine alkalinization. Rasburicase is a highly soluble IV recombinant form of urate oxidase, which can also be used to prevent or treat hyperuricemia. It acts by catalyzing the oxidation of uric

Table 2
Tumor lysis syndrome drug therapies

Drug	Dosing	Mechanism
Acetazolamide	Oral: 5 mg/kg/dose repeated 2-3 times during 24 h	Inhibits carbonic anhydrase, increased renal excretion of sodium, potassium, bicarbonate, and water. Urine alkalization decreases urate crystal precipitation.
Allopurinol	Oral: 600-800 mg/d in 2-3 divided doses IV: 200–400 mg/m^2/d (max 600 mg/d)	Xanthine analog; competitively inhibits xanthine oxidase, blocks the metabolism of hypoxanthine and xanthine to uric acid. Decreases the formation of new uric acid. Reduce dosage by 50% in the setting of renal insufficiency.
Rasburicase	Low-risk with baseline uric acid <7.5 mg/dL—rasburicase 0.10 mg/kg Intermediate risk with baseline uric acid ≤7.5 mg/dL—rasburicase 0.15 mg/kg High-risk baseline uric acid level > 7.5 mg/dL (450 mmol/L)— rasburicase 0.2 mg/kg	Catalyzes oxidation of uric acid to allantoin, which is more water soluble than uric acid and easily excreted.
Aluminum hydroxide	50–150 mg/kg/d divided every 4–6 h	Binds phosphate and bile salts to form an insoluble compound. Reduces serum phosphate levels. Risk of aluminum toxicity limits its use in renal failure
Mannitol	0.5–1 g IV bolus	Increases the osmotic pressure of glomerular filtrate, preventing reabsorption of water and electrolytes and increasing urinary output. Increases phosphate excretion

acid to allantoin, which is 5 to 10 times more soluble in urine than in uric acid. Rasburicase effectively decreases levels of uric acid, xanthine, and hypoxanthine by reducing existing pools and preventing further production of uric acid. Although simultaneous hyperhydration is recommended, rasburicase does not require concomitant urine alkalinization and, thereby, also encourages phosphate excretion.[14] Several studies have verified its safety in pediatric as well as adult patients.[16] It is contraindicated in the setting of glucose-6-phosphate dehydrogenase deficiency, pregnancy, methemoglobinemia, or previous allergy and has a known side effect of hemolytic anemia. The 2008 International Expert Panel on TLS has provided rasburicase dosing guidelines based on the level of risk for TLS and uric acid levels, which can be found in **Table 2**.[17] Several small studies demonstrated effective treatment and prophylaxis for TLS and noted a decreased incidence of renal failure with the use of rasburicase.[18] One study of 11 patients showed a drop in uric acid to normal levels with a single dose regimen.[19,20] Rasburicase has shown promising results for treatment and prophylaxis of TLS as well as prevention of TLS-induced renal failure, though more large-scale studies are needed.

Hyperphosphatemia may be treated with oral phosphate binders, such as aluminum hydroxide, with careful observation for aluminum toxicity in the renally impaired patient. Mannitol should be given only for hyperphosphatemia refractory to aluminum hydroxide in a well-hydrated patient.[21] Dialysis should be considered early, especially in the presence of hyperphosphatemia greater than 10 mg/dL, ARF, extreme potassium abnormalities, or a calcium-phosphate product greater than 50. The calcium-phosphate product can be easily calculated by multiplying the serum phosphate and total serum calcium levels. A level greater than 50 promotes calcium-phosphate deposition in renal tubules and will exacerbate underlying renal insufficiency.

TLS is a true oncologic emergency that is both preventable and amenable to treatment. Consultation with the patient's oncologist and admitting service is necessary to support the patient's ability to successfully complete chemotherapy and prevent the complications of TLS.

Nephrotoxic Drugs

Although aggressive treatment of malignancy is the cornerstone of successful outcomes, the available therapies carry their own risk profile. Many of the agents commonly used in the treatment of patients with malignancy, unfortunately, are known to carry a risk of nephrotoxicity. Chemotherapeutic agents are well known for their myriad side effects, and the agents most notable for causing renal dysfunction include mitomycin, gemcitabine, platinum compounds, methotrexate, and ifosfamide. Non-chemotherapeutic drugs commonly used in the treatment of patients with malignancy that are well known threats to renal function include cyclosporine, tacrolimus amino-glycosides, and amphotericin B.

Cyclosporine

Cyclosporine is the mainstay of treatment in BMT patients to prevent graft versus host disease. Cyclosporine is a well-known nephrotoxin whose acute toxicity is related to renal vasoconstriction, leading to decreased renal blood flow and reduced glomerular filtration. Long-term sequelae include interstitial fibrosis and arteriopathy. Correlation of serum levels to renal impairment is the rationale behind careful monitoring. In fact, studies have shown that in a well-monitored setting, cyclosporine is not a contributor to dialysis-dependent renal failure in BMT patients.[22-24] In the compromised patient, treatment includes discontinuation of the drug. Low-dose dopamine infusion (2 mcg/kg/min) has been reported to reverse renal dysfunction.[25]

Tacrolimus

Tacrolimus is another immunosuppressive used for prophylaxis of transplant rejection and for graft versus host disease. Nephrotoxicity is a known complication, and in a study of patients receiving stem cell transplants, more than half the patients doubled their Cr. Hemolytic uremic syndrome has also been described with tacrolimus use.[26]

Aminoglycosides

Gentamicin and other aminoglycosides are antibiotics commonly used in the treatment of life-threatening infections often encountered in the oncologic patient. Amino-glycosides are nephrotoxins associated with renal tubular damage manifested by proteinuria, oliguria, and azotemia. Careful serum level monitoring is tantamount, since levels more than the therapeutic range correlate with renal insufficiency. Particular drug combinations, such as gentamicin-cephalothin, that are well known to act synergistically in precipitating renal compromise should be avoided.[6]

Amphotericin B

Use of Amphotericin B is reserved for life-threatening fungal infections due to the high incidence of nephrotoxicity. Mechanisms of injury include renal vasoconstriction and direct tubular injury. Renal injury from Amphotericin B is dose related and cumulative. Fortunately, renal impairment is usually reversible with cessation of the drug.

Contrast Agents

Contrast agent nephropathy is one of the most common causes of renal failure in the cancer patient and one of the most avoidable. Typically, contrast agent-induced nephropathy is reversible and resolves within a few weeks without dialysis. Unfortunately, in cancer patients, particularly those with multiple myeloma, the damage can be irreversible and lead to chronic dialysis. As with all patients, vigilance before contrast infusion can prevent most renal compromise. Correction of pre-existing hypovolemia, pre- and postcontrast infusion hydration, and judicious dosing of contrast agent are all successful strategies to prevent nephropathy. For high-risk patients, such as those with multiple myeloma, consideration should be given for the use of nonionic, iso-osmolar contrast agents as well as a lower dose. Consultation with a radiologist can facilitate a cost-effective strategy to reserve the use for high-risk patients susceptible to injury. Protective use of N-acetyl cysteine may be considered, although solid evidence of benefit is yet to be established.[27] In the ED, the risk of IV contrast dye may be outweighed by the need to perform the appropriate radiographic study to diagnose life-threatening conditions.

Complications of Bone Marrow Transplant

In addition to immunosuppression with nephrotoxic drugs, BMT carries its own risk of renal complications. In the early phase following BMT, microangiopathy and graft versus host disease are etiologic causes for renal dysfunction along with drug toxicity, with a higher incidence in allogenic transplants. The most common time frame for the development of ARF following BMT is during the first 3 weeks. A unique hepatorenal-like syndrome has also been described and may be seen in up to 90% of post-BMT patients with ARF.[22] This syndrome, which is due to damage within the hepatic sinusoids, presents with jaundice and portal hypertension preceding the ARF, sodium retention with associated edema, a high blood urea nitrogen (BUN)/Cr ratio, mild hyponatremia, and hypotension.

Approximately 6 weeks post-BMT, TMA, which resembles the hemolytic-uremic syndrome, may also occur. This syndrome of nephritis, severe hypertension with associated neurologic complications, microangiopathic anemia and thrombocytopenia, and renal failure occur in 15% to 20% of patients. Although there are many possible causes for TMA, total-body irradiation appears to be the major culprit.[22] Patients undergoing allogenic transplants who receive higher doses of whole-body irradiation have a higher rate of renal dysfunction (up to 45%). Supportive therapy is the mainstay of care in these patients. Late renal complications occurring after 100 days or more post-BMT are most commonly drug related.[4]

POSTRENAL AZOTEMIA
ExtraRenal Obstruction

ARF secondary to obstruction is a less common etiology for renal compromise but often amenable to treatment. Obstruction may be due to cancers of the kidney, bladder, or prostate or due to abdominal metastasis. Although hydronephrosis is a common finding, it may be absent early in the course of obstruction or when obstruction is partial. Diagnosis is made by abdominal imaging, most commonly renal ultrasonography. Relief of obstruction can be provided with a ureteral stent or percutaneous nephrostomy. Recovery of renal function is dependent on the time course and severity of obstruction.[9]

IntraRenal Obstruction

The hallmark of intra-renal obstructive etiologies is cast nephropathy, which occurs in patients with multiple myeloma. ARF is a common presenting diagnosis in patients with multiple myeloma and may be caused by amyloidosis and glomerular infiltration with light chains in addition to cast nephropathy. Cast nephropathy can be precipitated by hypovolemia, sepsis, urinary pH more than 7, or hypercalciuria. Therapy involves hydration, elimination of nephrotoxic compounds, urine alkalinization in patient with Bence-Jones proteinuria, and correction of hypercalcemia. Other therapy includes alkylating agents with high-dose steroids.[8] Plasma exchange may have some theoretical benefit in clearing light chains, but no survival benefit or decrease in dialysis dependence has been demonstrated.[28]

MANAGEMENT

In the emergent treatment of the oncologic patient with renal dysfunction, it is important to help identify the underlying cause of renal dysfunction, as the treatment for the various insults is diverse. A detailed history outlining the course of the patient's disease, recent symptoms, concurrent illness, chemotherapeutic regimen, and other medication therapy is paramount in the care of these patients. An electrocardiogram can be used to quickly screen for the presence of hyperkalemia, and in the appropriate setting, a bedside ultrasound or bladder scan can identify acute urinary retention. Laboratory markers including BUN, Cr, serum electrolytes, magnesium, phosphate, calcium, and uric acid levels as well as a urinalysis are essential in the evaluation of the oncologic patient with renal dysfunction. It is also important to include appropriate drug levels if indicated for nephrotoxic drugs, such as cyclosporine, tacrolimus, and aminoglycosides. Studies with nephrotoxic contrast medium should be avoided in the presence of renal dysfunction. Consultation with oncology and nephrology should be sought, as the management of these patients can be very complex. The recognition of the etiology for renal dysfunction along with appropriate aggressive treatment can influence the prognosis for survivorship in the patient with malignancy.

Studies describe a survival rate of 35% to 65% in leukemic patients with renal failure. The large amount of variability relates to the inclusion or exclusion of patients undergoing chemotherapy, BMT, and the presence or absence of multiorgan failure in studied groups.[4,7,29] Mortality is at least 30%, but mortality rates can be much higher in ARF patients admitted to the intensive care unit. Factors associated with a poor prognosis are similar for all patients with renal failure and include advanced age, sepsis, need for mechanical ventilation, and other organ failure.[7] Mortality for ARF patients with these comorbidities approaches 100%.[30]

SUMMARY

ARF is associated with a poor prognosis in cancer patients. Prevention, proactive surveillance, and aggressive therapy are all effective strategies that can diminish its impact on the patient with malignancy. A multidisciplinary approach to care is essential to optimize outcomes.

REFERENCES

1. Alexanian R, Barlogie B, Dixon D. Renal failure in multiple myeloma. Arch Intern Med 1990;150:1693–5.
2. Blade J, Fernandez-Llama P, Bosch F, et al. Renal failure in multiple myeloma: presenting features and predictors of outcome in 94 patients from a single institution. Arch Intern Med 1998;158:1889–93.
3. Cordonnier C, Vernant JP, Brun B, et al. Acute promyelocyctic leukemia in 57 previously untreated patients. Cancer 1985;55:18–25.
4. Munker R, Hill U, Kolb H. Renal complications in acute leukemias. Haematologica 1998;83:416–21.
5. Augustson BM, Begum G, Dunn JA, et al. Early Mortality after diagnosis of multiple myeloma: analysis of patients entered onto the United Kingdom Medical Research Trials between 1980–2002. Medical Research Council Working Party. J Clin Oncol 2005;23(36):9219–26.
6. Eckman LN, Lynch EC. Acute renal failure in patients with acute leukemia. South Med J 1978;71(4):382–5.
7. Harris KPG, Hattersley JM, Feehally J, et al. Acute renal failure associated with hematologic malignancies: a review of 10 years experience. Eur J Haematol 1991;47:119–22.
8. Kastritis E, Anagnostopoulos A, Roussou M, et al. Reversibility of renal failure in newly diagnosed multiple myeloma patients treated with high dose dexamethasone containing regimes and the impact of novel agents. Haematologica 2007; 92:546–9.
9. Darmon M, Ciroldi M, Thiery G, et al. Clinical Review: Specific aspects of acute renal failure in cancer patients. Crit Care 2006;10:211. Available at: http://ccforum.com/content/10/2/211. Accessed September 15, 2008.
10. Da'as N, Polliack A, Cohen Y, et al. Kidney involvement and renal manifestations in non-Hodgkin's lymphoma and lymphocytic leukemia: a retrospective study in 700 patients. Eur J Haematol 2001;67:158–64.
11. Rifkin SI. Acute renal failure secondary to chronic lymphocytic leukemia: a case report. Medscape J Med 2008;10(3):67.
12. Montesinos P, Lorenzo I, Martín G, et al. Tumor lysis syndrome in patients with acute myeloid leukemia: identification of risk factors and development of a predictive model. Haematologica 2008;93(1):67–74.
13. Conger JD, Falk SA. Intrarenal dynamics in the pathogenesis and prevention of acute urate nephropathy. J Clin Invest 1977;59(5):786–93.
14. Yamaguchi T, Sugimoto T, Imai Y, et al. Successful treatment of hyperphosphatemic tumoral calcinosis with long-term acetazolamide. Bone 1995;16(4): 247S–50S.
15. Coiffier B, Riouffol C. Management of tumor lysis syndrome in adults. Expert Rev Anticancer Ther 2007;7(2):233–9.
16. Goldman SC, Holcenberg JS, Finlestein JZ, et al. A randomized comparison between Rasburicase and allopurinol in children with lymphoma or leukemia at high risk for tumor lysis. Blood 2001;97(10):2998–3003.
17. Coiffier B, Altman A, Pui CH, et al. Guidelines for the management of pediatric and adult tumor lysis syndrome: an evidence-based review. J Clin Oncol 2008; 26:2767–78.
18. Pui CH, Mahmoud HH, Wiley JM, et al. Recombinant Urate oxidase for the prophylaxis or treatment of hyperuricemia in patients with leukemia or lymphoma. J Clin Oncol 2001;19(3):697–704.

19. McDonnell AM, Lenz KL, Frei-Lahr DA, et al. Single-dose rasburicase 6 mg in the management of tumor lysis syndrome in adults. Pharmacotherapy 2006;26(6): 806–12.
20. Hummel M, Reiter S, Adam K, et al. Effective treatment and prophylaxis of hyperuricemia and impaired renal function in tumor lysis syndrome with low doses of rasburicase. Eur J Haematol 2007;80(4):331–6.
21. Razis E, Arlin ZA, Ahmed T, et al. Incidence and treatment of tumor lysis syndrome in patients with acute leukemia. Acta Haematol 1994;91(4):171–4.
22. Zager RA. Acute renal failure in the setting of bone marrow transplantation. Kidney Int 1994;46:1443–58.
23. Zager RA, O'Quigley J, Zager BK, et al. Acute renal failure following bone marrow transplantation: a retrospective study of 272 patients. Am J Kidney Dis 1989;13: 210–6.
24. Mihatsch MJ, Ryffel B. Renal side effects of cyclosporine A with special reference to autoimmune disease. Br J Dermatol 1990;122(Suppl 36):101–15.
25. Conte G, Dal Canton A, Sabbatini M. Acute cyclosporine renal dysfunction reversed by dopamine infusion in healthy subjects. Kidney Int 1989;36:1086–92.
26. Woo M, Przepiorka D, Ippoliti C. Toxicities of tacrolimus and cyclosporin A after allogeneic blood stem cell transplantation. Bone Marrow Transplant 1997;20: 1095–8.
27. Hoffman U, Fischereder M, Kruger B, et al. The value of N acetyl cysteine in the prevention of radiocontrast agent-induced nephropathy seems questionable. J Am Soc Nephrol 2004;15:407–10.
28. Clark WF, Stewart AK, Rock GA, et al. Canadian Apheresis Group. Plasma exchange when myeloma presents as acute renal failure: a randomized, controlled trial. Ann Intern Med 2005;143:774–84.
29. Lanore JJ, Brunet F, Pochard F, et al. Hemodialysis for acute renal failure in patients with hematologic malignancies. Crit Care Med 1991;19(30):346–51.
30. Lameire NH, Flombaum CD, Moreau D, et al. Acute renal failure in cancer patients. Ann Med 2005;37:13–25.

Radiation Therapy– Related Toxicity (Including Pneumonitis and Fibrosis)

Rahul R. Chopra, MD*, Jeffrey A. Bogart, MD

KEYWORDS

- Radiation therapy • Toxicity • Inflammation
- Corticosteroids • Endarteritis • Fibrosis

In the modern age of cancer therapy, multidisciplinary management has led to increasing rates of survivorship. Surgery, chemotherapy, and radiation therapy (RT) are often integrated to optimize the likelihood of local control and survival for a wide spectrum of malignancies. RT toxicity must be tempered with the desire to deliver intensive therapy with the goal of improving tumor control and cure. The differential diagnosis for many RT-related toxicities is extensive. Several factors can modulate RT-related toxicity, including ancillary treatments, such as surgery and chemotherapy, as well as the underlying nutritional and medical status of the patient. This article is designed to acquaint emergency medicine physicians with common toxic effects in patients undergoing RT.

THERAPEUTIC MECHANISM OF CLINICAL RADIATION THERAPY

The principal therapeutic beam in radiation oncology is the x-ray (or γ-ray), and it consists of a large number of photons, or "packets," of energy.[1] The absorption of energy from radiation in a biologic material may lead to excitation or to ionization within the atoms of the biologic tissue.[2] The raising of an electron in an atom or molecule to a higher energy level without actual ejection of the electron is called excitation. If the photon is of sufficient energy, ejection of 1 or more orbital electrons from the atom can occur, and this process is referred to as ionization. The radiation that causes this is referred to as ionizing radiation.[2] The most important characteristic of ionizing radiation is the localized release of large amounts of energy. The energy dissipated per ionizing event (33 eV) is more than enough to break strong chemical bonds. Charged particles, such as electrons, protons, and α-particles, are *directly* ionizing, whereas

Department of Radiation Oncology, State University of New York Upstate Medical University, 750 East Adams Street, Syracuse, NY 13210, USA
* Corresponding author.
E-mail address: choprar@upstate.edu (R.R. Chopra).

Emerg Med Clin N Am 27 (2009) 293–310
doi:10.1016/j.emc.2009.01.010
0733-8627/09/$ – see front matter © 2009 Elsevier Inc. All rights reserved.

emed.theclinics.com

uncharged particles, such as photons and neutrons, are *indirectly* ionizing.[1] Provided that charged particles have sufficient kinetic energy, they can directly disrupt the atomic structure of the biologic material through which they pass, creating chemical and biologic damage. Uncharged particles, with energy similar to photons, do not directly produce chemical and biologic damage themselves, but when they are absorbed in the material through which they pass, they give up their energy to produce fast-moving charged particles, known as free radicals, that are able to produce damage.

Conventional RT involves using x-rays to produce biologic damage. When a photon hits a water molecule in a cell, generation of a hydroxyl free radical occurs. It is estimated that two-thirds of the x-ray damage to DNA in mammalian cells is caused by the hydroxyl radical.[2] Damage to cellular DNA is the primary mechanism through which radiation is able to exert its therapeutic effect. When a cancer attempts to divide with a damaged genome, it undergoes a mitotic death.

RADIOBIOLOGICAL EFFECTS OF RADIATION THERAPY AT THE CELLULAR AND TISSUE LEVEL

RT is a local modality that generally causes toxicity limited to the area of treatment (with some caveats). The effects of RT on normal tissues generally result from the depletion of a cell population by cell killing. The cells of normal tissue are not independent units but rather form a complete integrated structure. Response to RT is governed by 3 main factors: (1) inherent cellular radiosensitivity, (2) kinetics of the tissue, and (3) organization of cells within the tissue. Visible damage to an organ becomes evident only if a sufficient proportion of cells are killed. As mentioned previously, cell death after irradiation occurs when cells try to divide. In tissues with rapid turnover, damage can become evident quickly—in a matter of hours (as in gastrointestinal [GI] mucosa) or days (skin). This gives rise to the concept of "early" responding tissues. "Late" responding tissues have toxicity that occurs after a delay of months or years and predominantly in slowly proliferating tissues, such as the lung, kidney, heart, liver, and the central nervous system (CNS).[3] Acute damage is generally repaired quickly secondary to rapid proliferation of underlying stem cells. Late effects, in contrast, may improve but never completely repair. A late effect generally results from a combination of vascular damage through radiation endarteritis in combination with a loss of parenchymal cells. Radiation endarteritis leads to significant atherosclerotic disease several years after initial therapy, in the areas that previously received RT. If an intensive radiation regimen is used with subsequent depletion of the stem-cell population below levels needed for tissue repair, an early reaction in a rapidly proliferating tissue may persist as a chronic injury. This is termed a consequential late effect.[3] An example of this would be necrosis or fibrosis of the skin that occur consequent to severe radiation dermatitis and acute ulceration.

Another concept that is important in understanding radiation toxicity is the idea of an underlying organ's makeup, namely its functional subunits. The tolerance of normal tissues to radiation is dependent on the ability of clonogenic tissue progenitor cells to maintain a sufficient number of differentiated cells that are appropriately structured to maintain organ function. The structural organization of a tissue is crucial in determining the relationship between survival of clonogenic progenitor cells and organ function versus failure. Structurally *defined* functional subunits can include the hepatic lobule, the renal nephron, or the pulmonary acinus. Structurally *undefined* functional units are seen in the cutaneous skin where re-epithelialization of a denuded area can occur either from surviving clonogens within the affected area or by migration from adjacent areas. In the case of organs such as the lung, liver, and kidney, a certain portion can be treated without significant dysfunction. The subunits in these tissues work in *parallel* to carry out the physiologic function. This is in contrast to *serial* tissues, such as the spinal cord, where disruption of a portion of the tissue affects all downstream activity.[3]

RT is generally given as a number of small doses on a daily basis, rather than one large fraction (although this does occur as well and is generally referred to as radiosurgery). Dividing a dose into a number of smaller doses, or fractions, allows normal tissues to be spared. This is due to repair of cellular damage that occurs each day. Normal cells typically have better repair mechanisms than those of cancer cells, and RT is used to exploit this difference. Prolonging overall treatment time and decreasing fraction size will generally decrease the severity of "early" effects. Increasing the dose of radiation per fraction to normal tissue may not affect the patient acutely but results in an increased risk of "late" effects several months to several years later.[3] A review of classically defined radiation tolerance is shown in **Table 1**. The TD 5/5 and TD 50/5 in **Table 1** refer to radiation doses that would be expected to cause a 5% or 50% rate of the given complication or toxicity at 5 years.

TOXICITY BY ORGAN SYSTEM
Skin and Soft Tissue Toxicity

Acute radiation toxicity of the skin generally has a time course of several days to weeks after beginning RT. Before the advent of modern megavoltage linear accelerators, acute skin toxicity was the most common dose-limiting factor. Clinical signs of acute radiation toxicity can include erythema, edema, and hyperpigmentation. At higher doses, both moist desquamation and dry desquamation can occur.[4] Management generally consists of cleansers, moisturizers, petrolatum-based products (for dry desquamation), topical steroids (somewhat controversial), wound cleaners/epithelial stimulants, and hydrocolloid dressings.[5] Skin reactions are typically self-limited and will resolve over a matter of a few weeks' time. In some cases with severe desquamation, topical burn medication such as silvadene cream may be required, and patients may need to be admitted for wound management and antibiotics for a potential superinfection.

Fibrosis is one of the most common chronic skin and soft tissue toxicities that occur in patients who have undergone RT, with a time course that begins several months to a few years after completing RT. This may occur in the absence of a severe acute skin reaction. The etiology is thought to be a characteristic RT-induced endarteritis with vascular and capillary damage. Chronic tissue hypoxia leads to fibroblast proliferation and eventual scarring and fibrosis of the affected tissue. As with any late effect, dose, volume, and RT fractionation can affect the eventual clinical outcome. Other factors such as previous surgical manipulation and underlying medical comorbidities, such as diabetes, hypertension, and vascular disease, can also affect tissue oxygenation and increase the prevalence of fibrosis. Fibrosis is generally permanent, and the severity may increase with further follow-up. Clinical signs can include cutaneous induration, lymphedema, joint restriction, ulcerations, atrophy, telangiectasia, and photosensitivity.[5] Skin and soft tissue necrosis is generally managed with supportive care. A combination of pentoxifylline (PTX) and vitamin E has been examined for treatment of fibrosis. Initial studies in swine models demonstrated an approximate 50% decrease in the dimensions of fibrosis.[6] This was confirmed in a small study of breast cancer patients given 800 mg/d of PTX and 1000 U/d of Vitamin E. A statistically significant regression in radiation-induced fibrosis was noted in patients taking both medications for 6 months. Nevertheless, the authors concluded that these results require confirmation in a larger study.[7] Longitudinal studies suggest that a long

Table 1
Normal tissue tolerance to therapeutic irradiation: clinical endpoints and possible management strategies

Organ	TD 5/5 (Dose in Gy)	TD 50/5 (Dose in Gy)	Clinical Endpoint	Management Considerations
Kidneys	23–50	28–40	Nephritis	Expectant/dialysis
Bladder	65–80	80–85	Bladder contracture/volume loss/refractory hematuria	Consider hyperbaric oxygen (HBO)
Bladder			Acute cystitis/spasm	Analgesics (eg, phenazopyridine) and/or antispasmodics (eg, oxybutynin)
Femoral head	52	65	Necrosis	—
Skin	55–70	70	Necrosis, ulceration	Wound/burn management (silvadene, antibiotics, skin grafting if severe)
Skin			Acute desquamation	Moisturizing creams, hydrocortisone cream, hydrogel wound dressing, consider empiric antibiotics
Bone (mandible)			Osteoradionecrosis	Surgical debridement, antibiotics, consider HBO
Oral mucosa	60	75	Ulceration, fibrosis, mucositis	Wound care, oral hygiene and baking soda mouthwash, gelclair, narcotics, topical anesthetics, consider empiric antifungal
Brain	45–60	60–75	Necrosis, infarction	Corticosteroids, mannitol, neurosurgical evaluation
Spinal cord	47–50	70	Myelitis, necrosis	HBO questionable, high-dose steroids questionable
Brachial plexus	60–62	75–77	Plexopathy, nerve damage	HBO questionable, high-dose steroids questionable, physical therapy

Structure			Toxicity	Management
External/middle ear	30–55	40–65	Acute/chronic serous otitis	Earwax removal (Debrox), pseudoephedrine, myringotomy in severe cases
Parotid	32	46	Xerostomia	Pilocarpine, artificial saliva, antibacterial mouthwash, dental gum
Lung	18–45	25–65	Pneumonitis	Corticosteroids, antibiotics
Heart	40–60	50–70	Pericarditis	Corticosteroids, nonsteroidal anti-inflammatory
Esophagus	55–60	68–72	Stricture, perforation	Dilation
Esophagus			Acute esophagitis	Oral anesthetic solutions (eg, viscous lidocaine + benadryl or sucralfate suspension), soft diet, consider empiric antifungal
Prostate			Urinary irritative/obstructive symptoms	Alpha-1 blocker, anti-inflammatory, phenazopyridine (caution with antispasmodics)
Stomach	50–60	65–70	Ulceration, perforation	Surgical management
Small intestine	40–50	55–60	Obstruction, perforation, fistula	Surgical management
Colon	45–55	55–65	Obstruction, perforation, fistula	Surgical management
Rectum	60	80	Proctitis	Mesalamine, sulfasalazine, sucralfate enema, steroid suppositories

Adapted from Emami B, Lyman J, Brown A, et al. Tolerance of normal tissue to therapeutic irradiation. Int J Radiat Oncol Biol Phys 1991;21(1):109–22; with permission.

duration of therapy (12–24 months) is required for maximal regression of fibrosis.[8] Hyperbaric oxygen (HBO) treatment may also be effective for soft tissue necrosis. In one review of 23 patients with soft tissue or bony necrosis of the chest wall, HBO was an important adjunct to surgical debridement, with or without flap placement, and improvement was noted in the majority of patients.[9]

Pulmonary Toxicity

The pulmonary toxic effects of RT can have devastating and longstanding consequences, and this risk must be considered during treatment planning for lung cancer, breast cancer, and other thoracic malignancies. Pulmonary toxicity often presents with an acute inflammatory phase, which may be self-limited and improve with supportive measures, although severe cases may prove fatal. The later onset of RT-related pulmonary fibrosis (PF), which includes fibroblast proliferation and the destruction of normal lung architecture, has more lasting consequences.

Acute pulmonary toxicity that occurs in a previously radiated lung is referred to as radiation pneumonitis (RP). RP generally occurs within 1 to 3 months following completion of RT.[10,11] The underlying etiology and pathophysiology of RP are related to a cytokine-mediated signal cascade with proinflammatory and profibrotic factors.[10,12] Some preclinical studies suggest a role for transforming growth factor beta (TGF-β) and interleukin-6 (IL-6) as well as other cytokines in the development of RP.[10,12,13] Important factors in determining the risk of RP include volume of lung irradiated, the dose per RT fraction (to functioning lung), and the use of concurrent or sequential chemotherapy. Although several metrics have been evaluated to predict for RP, the V20, or volume of lung receiving at least 20 Gy, is the most frequently used parameter. Baseline poor pulmonary capacity and smoking may predict an increased risk of RP.[14] Individualized biologic factors are important, and serum TGF-β levels may help identify patients at risk of RP. A study from Duke University was successfully able to escalate the RT dose in patients who had lower TGF-β levels.[15]

The diagnosis of RP is generally made with an appropriate clinical history in a patient who has undergone previous RT to the chest (ie, lung cancer, breast cancer, or lymphoma). The differential diagnosis includes infectious pneumonia, pulmonary embolism, and tumor recurrence.[10,12] The diagnosis of RP may be particularly challenging in lung cancer patients who are at risk for pulmonary compromise due to severe underlying pulmonary dysfunction. Clinical symptoms are nonspecific and include cough (nonproductive or productive of clear sputum), low-grade fever, dyspnea, fatigue, and pleuritic chest pain.[11,12] Physical examination may reveal crackles or a pleural rub. Imaging very early on in the course of RP may not show abnormalities. Ground-glass opacities that conform to the RT port[11] classically define RP, although this is not a consistent finding.[11,16] In some patients, a lymphocytic alveolitis involving both adjacent lobes in the ipsilateral lung as well as the contralateral lung has been described after undergoing RT.[16] Symptoms are similar to RP, but radiographically, more diffuse changes are noted. A typical example of acute RP is shown in **Fig. 1**.

Single-photon emission computed tomography ventilation and perfusion scans can detect regional RT-induced lung injury (RILI) even at modest doses of RT.[12,17] Pulmonary-function tests (PFTs) may be diminished, although the diffusing capacity of carbon monoxide is preferentially affected.[12,14,18] A restrictive pattern is likely to emerge on PFTs in the late fibrotic phase. The cornerstone of management of acute RP is the use of high-dose corticosteroids. A dose of 30 to 60 mg/d of prednisone or 16 to 20 mg/d of dexamethasone should be started once the diagnosis of RILI is established.[19] Others have advocated a prednisone dose of 1 mg/kg/d.[20] Steroids should be gradually tapered over a period of weeks (reduce daily dose by ~10 mg/wk)

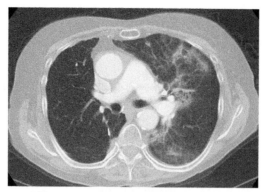

Fig. 1. Radiation pneumonitis: Computed tomographic (CT) scan.

to avoid flare-ups of RP.[19] Supplemental oxygen should be administered if indicated, and the differential diagnosis of infectious pneumonia must be considered. Symptoms of acute RP will generally improve over a matter of weeks to months with supportive management.

Several agents have shown promise in either reducing the risk of RP or treating RP. Clinical and preclinical studies have assessed captopril, cyclosporin, and PTX, amifostine, keratinocyte growth factor, and inhibitors of TGF-β. Amifostine has demonstrated variable effects in clinical studies but must be administered concurrently with thoracic RT to be effective.[21] Captopril, an angiotensin-converting enzyme inhibitor, is a thiol compound that can scavenge free radicals and stimulate IL-2. It has been found to reduce the incidence of RT-induced fibrosis in rats,[22] although extrapolation from this animal data suggests that much higher doses would be required for tissue protection than those administered for hypertension. A National Cancer Institute phase II randomized trial is currently underway to assess its efficacy.[20] Preclinical research involving a novel inhibitor of the TGF-β 1 receptor has demonstrated a decreased incidence in functional lung damage, inflammatory response, and serum TGF-β level.[22,23]

In the late setting, PF predominates.[9] PF generally occurs beyond 6 months.[10] The underlying pathophysiology is similar to fibrosis that occurs in other tissues, with pro-fibrotic cytokines, such as TGF-β IL-1 and IL-6, playing a role.[10,11] Chemotherapy with well-known agents, such as actinomycin D, adriamycin, bleomycin, busulfan, cyclophosphamide, and bis-chloronitrosourea, may exacerbate PF.[19] Many patients who previously received RT to the chest will have radiographic abnormalities, which may persist indefinitely, without exhibiting clinical symptoms. It is necessary to compare serial x-rays (if available) in patients who have a history of RT treatment to the chest to avoid misinterpreting chronic radiation changes as an acute process. An example of chronic radiation-induced fibrosis is shown in **Fig. 2**. Clinically significant RT-induced fibrosis may result in progressive chronic dyspnea;[11] however, there is no correlation between the extent of radiographic change and clinical symptoms.[10,11] Although current treatment is primarily supportive, ongoing research is evaluating the potential for several growth factor inhibitors to reverse PF.

Endobronchial (intraluminal) brachytherapy (EBBT) is generally used in patients who have relapsed and/or have persistent airway tumors. Patients often have already received full-dose external beam RT. Even in patients with recurrent lesions, EBBT is effective in relieving symptoms such as dyspnea, hemoptysis, and postobstructive pneumonitis.[24] Massive, sometimes fatal, hemoptysis is a feared severe complication

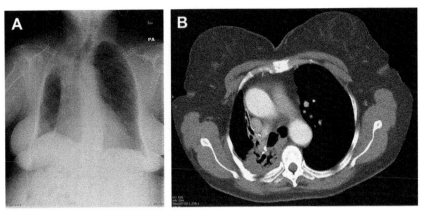

Fig. 2. Late radiation-associated PF and volume loss 7 y after treatment: (*A*) Chest x-ray. (*B*) Computed tomographic (CT) scan.

in patients undergoing EBBT. The largest series report fatal hemoptysis rates of 9% to 11%, and patients with tumors located in the main bronchi or upper lobes (possible close relationship to the pulmonary vasculature) were more likely to develop this complication.[24,25]

Stereotactic body radiation therapy (SBRT) involves the delivery of a few (< = 5) intense fractions of RT to a limited volume using advanced technologies. One of the most active areas of SBRT is in the treatment of patients with early stage nonsmall cell lung cancer who are unable to undergo surgical lobectomy. Although excellent rates of tumor control have been reported in several studies, there is an increased risk of severe pulmonary toxicity following treatment of centrally located (eg, peihilar) tumors due to resultant airway obstruction and atelectasis.[26] Radiographic changes are more severe than those seen with typical fractionated RT due to the ablative nature of SBRT. Another complication that is increasingly recognized in the treatment of peripheral lung lesions is rib pain and fracture. Treatment is typically supportive with analgesic medications.

Central Nervous System Toxicity

The risk of toxicity from CNS RT must be weighed against often dire consequences of tumor relapse in the brain. The underlying pathophysiology of acute neurocognitive change generally relates to radiation-induced disruption of the blood-brain barrier, which in and of itself may lead to increased toxicity when concurrent or adjuvant chemotherapy is used. The blood-brain barrier is disrupted secondary to endothelial cell damage, whereas glial cell damage can further contribute to neurotoxicity. Factors important in predicting long-term and short-term CNS toxic effects of RT include the RT volume, dose, fraction schedule, use of concurrent or sequential chemotherapy, and age of the patient (with extremes of age being more susceptible to toxicity).

Common acute side effects, which occur within a few weeks of beginning cranial RT, generally include mild fatigue, skin erythema, and alopecia. Radiation dermatitis, when it does occur, is usually mild and can be ameliorated with the use of topical oint- ments (eg, RadiaCare or Aquaphor). Nausea and headache are common in patients undergoing cranial RT and may be secondary to mild cerebral edema. The administra- tion of oral steroids (eg, Decadron in divided daily doses) and antinausea medication is usually effective management.

Patients who have elevated intracranial pressure (ICP) and received large-volume RT with a large fraction size (>3 Gy) are at risk for acute encephalopathy. Symptoms can include nausea and vomiting, headache, somnolence, fever, and focal neurologic deficits. It is important to realize that tumor-associated edema can cause many of the same side effects, and if symptomatic cerebral edema is present, corticosteroids may be indicated before beginning RT. In rare cases, cerebral herniation, or even death, can occur.[19]

A serous otitis media with mucosal vasodilation and Eustachian tube edema may occur after RT. In occasional cases, this may lead to tinnitus and high-frequency hearing loss requiring myringotomy tubes, and, in extreme cases, cochlear implants may be required.[27] Excessive cerumen buildup may occur within weeks to months after completing RT and can be treated with gentle earwax removal kits such as carbamide peroxide (Debrox) ear drops.

The somnolence syndrome includes symptoms of increased ICP, such as headache, nausea, vomiting, and irritability. The syndrome occurs most commonly in children who have previously undergone prophylactic whole-brain RT and is rare in adults.[28–30] There are no radiographic or laboratory findings that are specific to the diagnosis, and the syndrome is self-limited and usually resolves within 2 to 3 weeks. Corticosteroids may improve symptoms in patients with this syndrome, although their routine use is not recommended.[29]

Transient myelopathy may occur 2 to 4 months after spinal irradiation and may present with Lhermitte's sign, which consists of an unpleasant electric shock-like sensation that radiates down the spine and frequently into the limbs.[31] The symptoms are precipitated by flexion of the neck[19] and are thought to be due to transient demyelinization of the cord. Transient radiation myelopathy of the spinal cord is a clinical diagnosis without specific radiographic findings. The syndrome is self-limiting, lasting approximately 4 months on average, and does not require specific treatment and generally does not predict permanent neurologic compromise.

Radiation necrosis of the brain can occur months to years after RT. The etiology is vascular endothelial cell damage with resultant coagulative necrosis and demyelination secondary to chronic hypoxia.[32] Radiation necrosis generally develops in the high-dose region of RT, with symptoms dependent on the location of the lesion. Focal neurologic deficits and/or signs of increased ICP can occur. Conventional magnetic resonance imaging (MRI) findings include a contrast-enhancing mass with white-matter changes and/or edema. Magnetic resonance spectroscopy and fluorodeoxyglucose positron emission tomography imaging may help differentiate tumor recurrence from necrosis,[33] although pathologic confirmation may be necessary. The symptoms of radiation necrosis may be improved with corticosteroids and/or mannitol, although surgical decompression may be required. Experience treating radiation necrosis with anticoagulation and HBO is limited.[34,35]

Nonspecific, diffuse white matter changes occur in the vast majority of patients receiving conventional full-dose RT (in the case of gliomas, for example). Symptoms of leukoencephalopathy can occur in both children and adults and were first described in pediatric patients receiving prophylactic cranial RT and methotrexate for leukemia.[36] Initial symptoms may include lethargy and seizures and, in some cases, may progress to ataxia, overt confusion, dementia, and even death.[37] Differentiating adverse effects of cranial RT from the effects of the underlying malignancy can be difficult. Data from studies involving the use of methylphenidate as well as the acetylcholinesterase inhibitor donepezil suggest a benefit to both drugs in improving long-term NCF in patients who have undergone cranial RT.[38,39] The herb ginkgo biloba is also the focus of an ongoing study.[40]

Radiation myelopathy is an uncommon late complication of spinal RT. The initial symptoms can include paresthesias and sensory changes, such as a decrease in proprioception or temperature sensation. These symptoms begin anywhere from 9 to 15 months after completion of RT.[41] Progressive symptoms may include altered bowel and bladder function, lower-extremity weakness, hyperreflexia, and, in some cases, a Brown-Séquard syndrome. Chronic radiation myelopathy, in contrast to the transient form, is generally irreversible. Similar to transient myelopathy, this is a diagnosis of exclusion, and a thorough differential diagnosis, including tumor recurrence, demyelinating diseases, and neurotoxicity secondary to iatrogenic causes, should be considered. A spinal MRI with gadolinium may be helpful in establishing the diagnosis. An MRI may show cord atrophy or swelling, decreased intensity on T1 images, and increased intensity on the T2 sequence, frequently with contrast enhancement.[42] There is no definite evidence of an effective therapy for chronic progressive radiation myelopathy. Interventions such as HBO, heparin, and warfarin have been tried, but only anecdotal evidence exists for these measures.[34,43] Ongoing research is assessing the role of stimulating growth factors, including platelet-derived growth factor, insulin-like growth factor , vascular endothelial growth factor, and basic fibroblast growth factor, in treating radiation myelitis.[44]

Hypothalamic and pituitary dysfunction commonly occur in both children and adults following RT.[45] Growth hormone production is the most sensitive to RT, more so than adrenalcorticotropic hormone or thyrotropin-releasing hormone. Children are especially susceptible to effects of cranial RT, with a variable time course of endocrine dysfunction after receiving treatment.

Head and Neck Toxicity

RT is frequently employed as a primary treatment for early stage head and neck cancer (HNC) and often combined with chemotherapy for more advanced-stage tumors. Chemotherapy potentiates both the beneficial and toxic effects of RT. Severe acute reactions often expected during RT include mucositis, dysphagia, odynophagia, xerostomia, dermatitis, and voice changes. Tumor- and patient-related factors are important in predicting acute toxicity, and social factors (eg, current and/or prior history of alcohol/tobacco abuse, poor dentition, malnutrition) as well as underlying medical comorbidities may exacerbate toxicity.

Oral mucositis results from the radiation-induced mitotic death of basal cells of the oral mucosal epithelium.[46] The superficial layers of the oral mucosa are lost through normal physiologic sloughing. The subsequent denuding of the epithelium results in mucositis. Characteristic symptoms of mucositis may include erythema, edema, tenderness, pain, dysphagia, and hoarseness. Mucositis typically manifests 2 to 3 weeks after beginning RT. Oral hygiene, dietary modification, and maintenance of nutritional status are integral to the management of mucositis. Avoidance of spicy or acidic foods, caffeine, tobacco, and alcohol will help symptomatic patients. Prophylactic placement of a gastric feeding tube should be considered. Topical anesthetics, often in combination with diphenhydramine or an antacid, are used during treatment for patients who develop painful mucositis and esophagitis. A "BMX" solution consisting of 1% to 2% viscous lidocaine, diphenhydramine, and Maalox provides short-term relief for oral intake. Care should be taken with the use of lidocaine-containing solutions, since anesthetized mucosa is more susceptible to trauma. Topical non-Rx gel protectants, such as benzocaine (Oratect) gel and GELCLAIR bioadherent oral gel (Helsinn Healthcare SA, Lugano, Switzerland), may provide a temporary protective barrier for inflamed mucosa before eating. Opioids (long acting and short acting) may be indicated for pain control in patients with severe mucositis, and transdermal fentanyl can be considered in patients unable to swallow oral medication. Mucositis will generally begin to resolve within a few weeks following the completion of RT.

Xerostomia related to salivary gland dysfunction is a common permanent effect of RT for HNC. Oral hygiene is critical, because decreased saliva production increases the risk of dental decay. Patients should frequently rinse and gargle with a solution of baking soda, salt, and water to help break up thickened oral secretions. Saliva substitutes have met with variable success and acceptance, and some patients will routinely carry a bottle of water with them. Amifostine, a sulfhydryl agent, is a free radical scavenger that has been shown to reduce the incidence of acute and chronic xerostomia in patients receiving conventional RT as well as chemoradiation for HNC.[47,48] Pilocarpine, a cholinergic agent, has also been examined as an agent to reduce xerostomia. It is generally given 5 mg 3 times a day during RT and thereafter. In one study, there was an increased rate of salivary function in the pilocarpine-treated group compared with that in the placebo, but the benefit on quality of life was unclear.[49]

Patients undergoing RT for HNC are prone to develop oral candidiasis, which can exacerbate mucositis.[46] Treatment of oral candidiasis can be accomplished through either the use of topical antifungal medication (eg, Nystatin "swish and swallow") or systemic antifungal medication (eg, fluconazole), which may be better tolerated in patients experiencing severe mucositis.

The unilateral blood supply to each half of the mandible can predispose patients to osteoradionecrosis (ORN). ORN typically presents within 3 years after completion of RT for HNC. ORN can present with a variety of symptoms, including pain, loss of sensation, fistula, halitosis, trismus, pathologic fracture, or infection. The diagnosis of ORN generally relies on clinical examination of chronically exposed bone. Radiographic findings include decreased bone density and pathologic fractures. The incidence of ORN based on retrospective studies ranges from 0.4% to 56%, with one of the largest series reporting an incidence of 8.2%.[50] The most common location for ORN is the body of mandible. Tooth extractions following RT are a common precipitant to ORN,[50] and HBO protocols may be considered before extraction in patients at risk.[46] Mild ORN is generally managed conservatively with debridement, therapeutic ultrasound, and antibiotics.[51] When there is extensive bone and soft tissue necrosis, radical resection with immediate microvascular reconstruction is indicated.[52] HBO is generally recommended for the management of ORN, in that it increases oxygenation of irradiated tissue, promotes angiogenesis, enhances osteoblast repopulation, and fibroblast function.[46] If surgery is used to manage ORN, traditionally, 10 dives of postsurgical HBO were recommended.[53] More recent protocols generally call for 30 preoperative HBO sessions at 2.4 atm for 90 minutes each, followed by 10 treatments after surgery.[54] Before HBO therapy was available, reconstruction of previously irradiated mandibular tissue in patients with oropharyngeal and other head and neck tumors was often unsuccessful, with complications, including osteonecrosis, soft tissue radionecrosis, mucositis, dermatitis, and laryngeal radionecrosis, developing in 50% to 60% of patients. With HBO, success rates of up to 93% have been reported among selected patients.[55] In severe cases of ORN, partial mandibulectomy may be required.

Dysphagia and pharyngeal dysfunction are to be expected in patients receiving chemotherapy and RT in HNC. Radiation of the oropharynx can lead to edema, fibrosis, and, in rare cases, pharyngeal stenosis. One study examined serial swallowing studies (fluoroscopy and esophagograms) performed pretherapy, 1 to 3 months post-RT and 6 to 12 months post-RT. Post-treatment changes included reduced inversion of the cricopharyngeal muscle and laryngeal closure, promoting aspiration.[54]

Oropharyngeal strictures can be treated with balloon dilation, but they frequently recur. Severe pharyngeal/laryngeal edema that develops during a course of RT can interfere with respiration in extreme cases and may require tracheostomy.[55] Hoarseness may result from RT to the laryngeal structures and generally improves with time, although continued smoking after treatment is associated with persistent hoarseness.[56]

Toxic Effects of Abdominal and Pelvic Radiotherapy

The liver may be irradiated during treatment of lower-lobe lung cancers, esophageal tumors, stomach cancer, pancreatic malignancies, and lymphomas, in addition to primary liver tumors. RT-associated liver toxicity may present similarly to hepatitis with vague right upper quadrant abdominal pain progressing to hepatomegaly and ascites. Anicteric ascites generally occurs a few months after RT, although the onset can occur more rapidly after chemoradiation.[19] Alkaline phosphatase is usually increased in radiation hepatopathy. Chronic hepatitis and cirrhosis associated with RT are mediated by TGF-β, similar to radiation-associated PF.[57] The characteristic lesion seen in late radiation hepatopathy is central venous occlusive disease, which is characterized by retrograde congestion on liver biopsy. Veno-occlusive lesions can appear as early as 2.5 months after a patient undergoes RT. The differential diagnosis includes other causes of liver disease, such as infectious hepatitis, metastatic disease, and drug-induced hepatitis. Treatment is primarily supportive, although transplant may be considered in select cases of severe radiation hepatopathy.

The small and large intestine are vulnerable portions of the GI tract and can undergo radiation-associated enteritis. Acute GI symptoms that occur within a few weeks of starting RT include increased stool frequency and loss of form, with eventual diarrhea. This is generally self-limiting and occurs as the result of acute mucosal changes after the initiation of RT. These effects may be exacerbated by the coadministration of chemotherapy agents. The mucosa is rapidly renewed, limiting the duration of these acute effects. Gentle use of antidiarrheals can be considered in addition to dietary modification. Late effects of the GI tract, including stricture and ulceration, can occur secondary to radiation endarteritis and chronic ischemia. Ulceration and infarction necrosis can occur with rapid obliteration of the vessels, whereas fibrosis, strictures, and fistulas may form due to more gradual narrowing of the finer vasculature. Surgical handling of irradiated bowel must be performed cautiously due to the tenuous blood supply to limit further vascular dysfunction and injury. The differential diagnosis must include small-bowel obstruction in patients with prior abdominal surgery, whether or not RT has been given.

Acute radiation-associated proctitis is generally self-limiting, with symptoms such as diarrhea, rectal urgency, and, rarely, bleeding, resolving within a few months.[58] Chronic or late radiation proctitis generally occurs 1 to 2 years after undergoing RT and is due to epithelial atrophy and fibrosis associated with the obliterative "endarteritis" seen in other late radiation toxicity syndromes. Symptoms associated with chronic radiation proctitis include diarrhea, obstructed defecation (secondary to stricture development), bleeding, tenesmus, and, occasionally, fecal incontinence. Diagnosis of chronic radiation proctitis is based on the clinical history, confirmed with findings found on colonoscopy or sigmoidoscopy. Changes to the mucosa can include pallor with friability and telangiectasias.[59] Mucosal biopsies can assess for other causes of proctitis such as inflammatory bowel disorders, although they must be performed with the utmost care, as radiated tissue is more prone to fistula formation and chronic nonhealing ulcerations.[60] Treatment should be directed at symptom management. Dietary assessment is critical, and the routine use of stool softeners and/or fiber additives may be valuable in patients suffering from constipation. In patients with mild symptoms, such as a small amount of intermittent rectal bleeding, anti-inflammatory suppositories (eg, hydrocortisone, mesalamine) may be beneficial. Symptoms can resolve spontaneously in up to a third of patients.[61] Refractory rectal bleeding should be assessed by colonoscopy to assess for other causes. Sulfasalazine has also been used either in oral or enema preparations with some success. Steroids, such as prednisolone, that have been added to these preparations have demonstrated further efficacy.[62] Topical sucralfate (given twice a day as an enema) also shows some efficacy in small clinical studies and may be more efficacious than combination sulfasalazine/prednisolone.[62]

Acute genitourinary effects of RT to the bladder and urethra include urinary frequency, urgency, and irritation. These effects are exacerbated when concomitant chemotherapy is used. Incontinence is rarely observed in the acute period in patients who were continent before the initiation of therapy. General management includes urinary anesthetic agents and antispasmotics. Urinary tract infections may coexist and should be considered in cases of persistent or refractory symptoms. Dietary modification, particularly with the elimination of caffeine and alcohol, may help to minimize symptoms. In men who have been treated for prostate cancer with brachytherapy, there is a 5% to 15% risk of urinary retention due to prostate edema.[63] If possible, men should be taught how to perform intermittent self-catheterization rather than having an indwelling catheter. Urinary retention will generally resolve within a matter of weeks. Care should be taken to assess amount of residual urine in the bladder, as the administration of antispasmodics (eg, oxybutynin [Ditropan]) may precipitate urinary retention. Medication with alpha blockers (eg, tamsulosin [Flomax]) should be considered in men who have obstructive symptoms. Transurethral resection of the prostate after RT is associated with an increased risk of incontinence and should only be considered in men who are refractory to conservative measures. Acute urinary irritative symptoms generally resolve (or greatly improve) within 3 to 6 weeks following the completion of external beam RT but may persist for several months in men treated with permanent seed implant.

Late genitourinary complications of RT include persistent irritative voiding symptoms. Urinary incontinence may be precipitated or exacerbated, particularly in men who are postprostatectomy. Severe late radiation cystitis and hematuria may occur in 3% to 5% of patients. This requires evaluation by cystoscopy, as hematuria may also signify the presence of bladder cancer recurrence. Moreover, men who have received RT for prostate cancer are at increased risk for developing secondary bladder cancer. Hematuria that is refractory to conservative measures can be effectively treated with HBO. In one study of 57 patients with radiation-induced hemorrhagic cystitis (mean time, 48 months from completion of RT), 86% had either complete resolution or marked improvement after HBO.[64] Urethral stricture and bladder neck contracture occur in less than 5% of patients, but the risk is increased in patients treated with combined surgery and RT. Treatment with outpatient urethral dilation is generally successful in alleviating symptoms, although repeat dilations may be necessary.

Cardiac Toxicity

A spectrum of cardiac injury can occur when the heart is irradiated. Late effects are most common due to radiation-induced vascular damage and endarteritis. Acute effects, such as pericarditis, may be observed after treatment of a substantial volume of the entire heart, such as in selected cases of Hodgkin's lymphoma (HL), but this is relatively uncommon. Long-term effects include coronary artery disease (CAD), cardiomyopathy, valvular damage, and dysrhythmias. These effects generally manifest years to decades after the original course of RT. CAD may appear 10 to 15 years after RT but is also affected by the patient's underlying cardiac risk factors, including obesity, diabetes, smoking, hypertension, and family history. High-risk populations include those with breast cancer and HL, many of whom were treated at a young enough age to manifest chronic radiation toxicity several years later.

The hallmarks of late radiation-associated cardiotoxicity include diffuse fibrosis of the myocardial interstitium with narrowing of the arterial and capillary lumens. Eventually, the number of capillaries is reduced relative to the number of myocytes, leading to ischemia, cell death, and replacement with collagen and fibrin.[65] CAD results from injury to the intima of the cardiac endothelium in a cascade of events that is typical of atherosclerosis, including deposition of platelets and myofibroblasts along with replacement of the damaged intima.[65] Fibrosis can occur in the cusp and/or leaflets of the valves as well as the wall of the ventricles, affecting cardiac compliance and contractility.[66] Dysrhythmias can arise when fibrosis occurs within the conduction system.[67] HL patients who have been treated with RT have an increased risk of valvular heart disease.[68] Mortality from myocardial infarction is also increased in patients with HL, mainly in those who were treated with anthracycline-based chemotherapy or supradiaphragmatic RT.[69–71]

SUMMARY

Radiation oncologists and emergency department physicians must be familiar with the underlying pathophysiology of RT-induced normal tissue toxicity, particularly in the context of multimodality therapy. Although most acute toxicities will be managed by the oncology team, many patients presenting to the emergency department will have a history of cancer treatment including RT. A better appreciation and understanding of the acute and late toxicities associated with RT will help improve the medical decision making in these patients. Advances in radiation oncology technology coupled with an improved understanding of the underlying biology of toxic reactions should result in fewer severe complications in the future.

REFERENCES

1. Khan FM. Interactions of ionizing radiation. In: The Physics of radiation therapy. Philadelphia: Lippincott Williams & Wilkins; 2003. p. 59–61.
2. Hall EJ, Giaccia EJ. Physics and chemistry of radiation absorption. In: Radiobiology for the radiologist. Philadelphia: Lippincott Williams & Wilkins; 2006. p. 5–14.
3. Hall EJ, Giaccia EJ. Clinical response of normal tissues. In: Radiobiology for the radiologist. Philadelphia: Lippincott Williams & Wilkins; 2006. p. 327–44.
4. Goodman M, Hilderly LJ, Purl S. Integumentary and mucous membrane alterations. In: Groenwald SL, Goodman M, Yarbro CH, editors. Cancer nursing principles and practice. 4th edition. Boston (MA): Jones and Bartlett; 1997. p. 768–822.
5. Wood G, Casey L, Trotti A. Skin changes. In: Small W, Woloschak GE, editors. Radiation toxicity: a practical guide. New York: Springer Science; 2006. p. 170–81.
6. Lefaix JL, Delanian S, Vozenin MC, et al. Striking regression of subcutaneous fibrosis induced by high doses of gamma rays using a combination of pentoxifylline and alpha-tocopherol: an experimental study. Int J Radiat Oncol Biol Phys 1999;43(4):839–47.

7. Delanian S, Porcher R, Balla-Mekias S, et al. Randomized, placebo-controlled trial of combined pentoxifylline and tocopherol for regression of superficial radiation-induced fibrosis. J Clin Oncol 2003;21(13):2545–50.

8. Delanian S, Porcher R, Rudant J, et al. Kinetics of response to long-term treatment combining pentoxifylline and tocopherol in patients with superficial radiation-induced fibrosis. J Clin Oncol 2005;23(34):8570–9.

9. Feldmeier JJ, Heimbach RD, Davolt DA, et al. Hyperbaric oxygen as an adjunctive treatment for delayed radiation injury of the chest wall: a retrospective review of twenty-three cases. Undersea Hyperb Med 1995;22(4): 383–93.

10. Chen Y, Williams J, Ding I, et al. Radiation pneumonitis and early circulatory cytokine markers. Semin Radiat Oncol 2002;12(1 Suppl 1):26–33.

11. Monson JM, Stark P, Reilly JJ. Clinical radiation pneumonitis and radiographic changes after thoracic radiation therapy for lung carcinoma. Cancer 1998; 82(5):842–50.

12. Marks LB, Yu X, Vujaskovic Z, et al. Radiation-induced lung injury. Semin Radiat Oncol 2003;13(3):333–45.

13. Anscher MS, Kong FM, Andrews K, et al. Plasma transforming growth factor beta1 as a predictor of radiation pneumonitis. Int J Radiat Oncol Biol Phys 1998;41(5):1029–35.

14. Smith LM, Mendenhall NP, Cicale MJ, et al. Results of a prospective study evaluating the effects of mantle irradiation on pulmonary function. Int J Radiat Oncol Biol Phys 1989;16(1):79–84.

15. Anscher MS, Marks LB, Shafman TD, et al. Risk of long-term complications after TFG-beta1-guided very-high-dose thoracic radiotherapy. Int J Radiat Oncol Biol Phys 2003;56(4):988–95.

16. Arbetter KR, Prakash UB, Tazelaar HD, et al. Radiation-induced pneumonitis in the "nonirradiated" lung. Mayo Clin Proc 1999;74(1):27–36.

17. Rodrigues G, Lock M, D'Souza D, et al. Prediction of radiation pneumonitis by dose - volume histogram parameters in lung cancer–a systematic review. Radiother Oncol 2004;71(2):127–38.

18. Brady LW, Germon PA, Cander L. The effects of radiation therapy on pulmonary function in carcinoma in the Lung. Radiology 1965;85:130–4.

19. Constine LS, Milano MT, Friedman D, et al. Late effects of cancer treatment on normal tissues. In: Halperin EC, Perez CA, Brady LW, editors. Perez and Brady's principles and practice of radiation oncology. 5th edition. Philadelphia: Lippincott Williams & Wilkins; 2007. p. 320–55.

20. Bradley J, Movsas B. Radiation pneumonitis and esophagitis in thoracic irradiation. In: Small W, Woloschak GE, editors. Radiation toxicity: a practical guide. New York: Springer Science; 2006. p. 42–53.

21. Komaki R, Lee JS, Milas L, et al. Effects of amifostine on acute toxicity from concurrent chemotherapy and radiotherapy for inoperable non-small-cell lung cancer: report of a randomized comparative trial. Int J Radiat Oncol Biol Phys 2004;58(5):1369–77.

22. Ward WF, Molteni A, Tsao CH. Radiation-induced endothelial dysfunction and fibrosis in rat lung: modification by the angiotensin converting enzyme inhibitor CL242817. Radiat Res 1989;117(2):342–50.

23. Anscher MS, Thrasher B, Zgonjanin L, et al. Small molecular inhibitor of transforming growth factor-beta protects against development of radiation-induced lung injury. Int J Radiat Oncol Biol Phys 2008;71(3):829–37.

24. Kelly JF, Delclos ME, Morice RC, et al. High-dose-rate endobronchial brachytherapy effectively palliates symptoms due to airway tumors: the 10-year M.D. Anderson cancer center experience. Int J Radiat Oncol Biol Phys 2000;48(3): 697–702.

25. Ozkok S, Karakoyun-Celik O, Goksel T, et al. High dose rate endobronchial brachytherapy in the management of lung cancer: Response and toxicity evaluation in 158 patients. Lung Cancer 2008;62(3):326–33.

26. Timmerman R, McGarry R, Yiannoutsos C, et al. Excessive toxicity when treating central tumors in a phase II study of stereotactic body radiation therapy for medically inoperable early-stage lung cancer. J Clin Oncol 2006;24(30):4833–9.

27. Jereczek-Fossa BA, Zarowski A, Milani F, et al. Radiotherapy-induced ear toxicity. Cancer Treat Rev 2003;29(5):417–30.

28. Freeman JE, Johnston PG, Voke JM. Somnolence after prophylactic cranial irradiation in children with acute lymphoblastic leukaemia. Br Med J 1973;4:523.

29. Uzal D, Ozyar E, Hayran M, et al. Reduced incidence of the somnolence syndrome after prophylactic cranial irradiation in children with acute lymphoblastic leukemia. Radiother Oncol 1998;48:29.

30. Schultheiss T, Kun L, Ang K, et al. Radiation response of the central nervous system. Int J Radiat Oncol Biol Phys 1995;31:1093.

31. Jones AM. Transient radiation myelopathy. Br J Radiol 1964;37(727):744.

32. Burger PC, Mahley MS Jr, Dudka L, et al. The morphologic effects of radiation administered therapeutically for intracranial gliomas: a postmortem study of 25 cases. Cancer 1979;44(4):1256–72.

33. Henry RG, Vigneron DB, Fischbein NJ, et al. Comparison of relative cerebral blood volume and proton spectroscopy in patients with treated gliomas. AJNR Am J Neuroradiol 2000;21(2):357–66.

34. Glantz MJ, Burger PC, Friedman AH, et al. Treatment of radiation-induced nervous system injury with heparin and warfarin. Neurology 1994;44(11):2020–7.

35. Chuba PJ, Aronin P, Bhambhani K, et al. Hyperbaric oxygen therapy for radiation-induced brain injury in children. Cancer 1997;80(10):2005–12.

36. Price RA, Jamieson PA. The central nervous system in childhood leukemia. II. Subacute leukoencephalopathy. Cancer 1975;35(2):306–18.

37. Frytak S, Shaw JN, O'Neill BP, et al. Leukoencephalopathy in small cell lung cancer patients receiving prophylactic cranial irradiation. Am J Clin Oncol 1989;12(1):27.

38. Mulhern RK, Khan RB, Kaplan S, et al. Short-term efficacy of methylphenidate: a randomized, double-blind, placebo-controlled trial among survivors of childhood cancer. J Clin Oncol 2004;22(23):4795–803.

39. Shaw EG, Rosdhal R, D'Agostino RB, et al. Phase II study of donepezil in irradiated brain tumor patients: effect on cognitive function, mood, and quality of life. J Clin Oncol 2006;24(9):1415–20.

40. Le Bars PL, Katz MM, Berman N. A placebo-controlled, double-blind, randomized trial of an extract of ginkgo biloba for dementia. JAMA 1997;278:1327–32.

41. Schultheiss TE, Higgins EM, El-Mahdi AM. The latent period in clinical radiation myelopathy. Int J Radiat Oncol Biol Phys 1984;10(7):1109–15.

42. Wang PY, Shen WC, Jan JS. Serial MRI changes in radiation myelopathy. Neuroradiology 1995;37(5):374–7.

43. Luk KH, Baker DG, Fellows CF. Hyperbaric oxygen after radiation and its effect on the production of radiation myelitis. Int J Radiat Oncol Biol Phys 1978;4(5–6): 457–9.

44. Andratschke NH, Nieder C, Price RE, et al. Potential role of growth factors in diminishing radiation therapy neural tissue injury. Semin Oncol 2005;32(2 Suppl 3): S67–70.

45. Constine LS, Woolf PD, Cann D, et al. Hypothalamic-pituitary dysfunction after radiation for brain tumors. N Engl J Med 1993;328(2):87–94.

46. Blanco AI, Chao C. Management of radiation-induced head and neck injury. In: Small W, Woloschak GE, editors. Radiation toxicity: a practical guide. New York: Springer Science; 2006. p. 23–39.

47. Büntzel J, Küttner K, Fröhlich D, et al. Selective cytoprotection with amifostine in concurrent radiochemotherapy for head and neck cancer. Ann Oncol 1998;9(5): 505–9.

48. Wasserman TH, Brizel DM, Henke M, et al. Influence of intravenous amifostine on xerostomia, tumor control, and survival after radiotherapy for head-and-neck cancer: 2-year follow-up of a prospective, randomized, phase III trial. Int J Radiat Oncol Biol Phys 2005;63(4):985–90.

49. Fisher J, Scott C, Scarantino CW. Phase III quality-of-life study results: impact on patients' quality of life to reducing xerostomia after radiotherapy for head-and-neck cancer–RTOG 97-09. Int J Radiat Oncol Biol Phys 2003;56(3):832–6.

50. Reuther T, T Schuster T, Mende U. Osteoradionecrosis of the jaws as a side effect of radiotherapy of head and neck tumour patients—a report of a thirty year retrospective review. Int J Oral Maxillofac Surg 2003;32:289–95.

51. Wong JK, Wood RE, McLean M. Conservative management of osteoradionecrosis. Oral Surg Oral Med Oral Pathol Oral Radiol Endod 1997;84(1):16–21.

52. Shaha AR, Cordeiro PG, Hidalgo DA, et al. Resection and immediate microvascular reconstruction in the management of osteoradionecrosis of the mandible. Head Neck 1997;19(5):406–11.

53. Marx RE, Ames JR. The use of hyperbaric oxygen therapy in bony reconstruction of the irradiated and tissue-deficient patient. J Oral Maxillofac Surg 1982;40(7): 412–20.

54. Tibbles PM, Edelsberg JS. Hyperbaric Oxygen Therapy. N Engl J Med 1996; 334(25):1642–8.

55. Hart GB, Mainous EG. The treatment of radiation necrosis with hyperbaric oxygen (OHP). Cancer 1976;37:2580–5.

56. Eisbruch A, Lyden T, Bradford CR, et al. Objective assessment of swallowing dysfunction and aspiration after radiation concurrent with chemotherapy for head-and-neck cancer. Int J Radiat Oncol Biol Phys 2002;53:23–8.

57. Lee HJ, Zelefsky MJ, Kraus DH, et al. Long-term regional control after radiation therapy and neck dissection for base of tongue carcinoma. Int J Radiat Oncol Biol Phys 1997;38(5):995–1000.

58. Verdonck-de Leeuw IM, Keus RB, Hilgers FJ, et al. Consequences of voice impairment in daily life for patients following radiotherapy for early glottic cancer: voice quality, vocal function, and vocal performance. Int J Radiat Oncol Biol Phys 1999;44(5):1071–8.

59. Anscher MS, Peters WP, Reisenbichler H, et al. Transforming growth factor beta as a predictor of liver and lung fibrosis after autologous bone marrow transplantation for advanced breast cancer. N Engl J Med 1993;328(22):1592–8.

60. Babb RR. Radiation proctitis: a review. Am J Gastroenterol 1996;91(7):1309–11.

61. O'Brien PC, Hamilton CS, Denham JW, et al. Spontaneous improvement in late rectal mucosal changes after radiotherapy for prostate cancer. Int J Radiat Oncol Biol Phys 2004;58(1):75–80.

62. Chrouser KL, Leibovich BC, Sweat SD, et al. Urinary fistulas following external radiation or permanent brachytherapy for the treatment of prostate cancer. J Urol 2005;173(6):1953–7.

63. Gilinsky NH, Burns DG, Barbezat GO, et al. The natural history of radiation-induced proctosigmoiditis: an analysis of 88 patients. QJM 1983;52(205):40–53, Winter.

64. Kochhar R, Patel F, Dhar A, et al. Radiation-induced proctosigmoiditis. Prospective, randomized, double-blind controlled trial of oral sulfasalazine plus rectal steroids versus rectal sucralfate. Dig Dis Sci 1991;36(1):103–7.

65. Bucci J, Morris WJ, Keyes M, et al. Predictive factors of urinary retention following prostate brachytherapy. Int J Radiat Oncol Biol Phys 2002;53(1):91–8.

66. Corman JM, McClure D, Pritchett R, et al. Treatment of radiation induced hemorrhagic cystitis with hyperbaric oxygen. J Urol 2003;169(6):2200–2.

67. Cuzick J, Stewart H, Rutqvist L, et al. Cause-specific mortality in long-term survivors of breast cancer who participated in trials of radiotherapy. J Clin Oncol 1994;12(3):447–53.

68. Hardenbergh PH, Munley MT, Bentel GC, et al. Cardiac perfusion changes in patients treated for breast cancer with radiation therapy and doxorubicin: preliminary results. Int J Radiat Oncol Biol Phys 2001;49(4):1023–8.

69. Orzan F, Brusca A, Gaita F, et al. Associated cardiac lesions in patients with radiation-induced complete heart block. Int J Cardiol 1993;39(2):151–6.

70. Hull MC, Morris CG, Pepine CJ, et al. Valvular dysfunction and carotid, subclavian, and coronary artery disease in survivors of Hodgkin lymphoma treated with radiation therapy. JAMA 2003;290(21):2831–7.

71. Swerdlow AJ, Higgins CD, Smith P, et al. Myocardial infarction mortality risk after treatment for Hodgkin disease: a collaborative British cohort study. J Natl Cancer Inst 2007;99(3):206–14.

Emergencies Related to Cancer Chemotherapy and Hematopoietic Stem Cell Transplantation

David E. Adelberg, MD[a],*, Michael R. Bishop, MD[b]

KEYWORDS

- Chemotherapy • Stem cell transplant • Neutropenia • Anemia
- Cardiotoxicity • Graft-versus-host disease

With the widespread use of outpatient therapy for various malignant diseases, it is increasingly likely that emergency department (ED) physicians will encounter patients receiving one of a multitude of different cancer therapies, from traditional chemotherapy to the newer biologic agents and targeted therapies, used either alone or in combination. Patients receiving systemic cancer therapy are at risk for a variety of toxicities, ranging from mild nausea and vomiting to severe symptomatic cardiotoxicity. It is important for the ED physician to be aware of the most commonly encountered complications of cancer therapy, thus allowing optimal treatment of this cohort of patients.

CHEMOTHERAPY-RELATED COMPLICATIONS
Nausea and Vomiting

Cancer patients receiving chemotherapy are at risk not only for acute emesis, defined as occurring within the first 1 to 2 hours of chemotherapy administration, but also delayed emesis, which may occur more than 24 hours following completion of treatment

This work was supported by the Center for Cancer Research, National Cancer Institute, Intramural Research Program.

[a] Medical Oncology Branch, National Cancer Institute, 10 Center Drive, CRC/Room 12N226, Bethesda, MD 20892, USA

[b] Experimental Transplantation and Immunology Branch, National Cancer Institute, 10 Center Drive, CRC/Room 4-3152, Bethesda, MD 20892, USA

* Corresponding author.

E-mail address: adelbergd@mail.nih.gov (D.E. Adelberg).

Emerg Med Clin N Am 27 (2009) 311–331
doi:10.1016/j.emc.2009.01.005
0733-8627/09/$ – see front matter. Published by Elsevier Inc.

administration.[1,2] It is this delayed phenomenon that the ED physician will most likely encounter.

Most chemotherapy regimens with a moderate to high intrinsic emetogenicity are accompanied by regularly scheduled, prophylactic antiemetics, especially in the first 48 to 72 hours post-treatment. Chemotherapeutic agents with a greater than 90% likelihood of inducing emesis include cisplatin, mechlorethamine, streptozocin, cyclophosphamide (>1500 mg/m^2), carmustine (bis-chloronitrosourea), dacarbazine, and dactinomycin. Drugs with a moderate level of emesis induction (between 30% and 90% frequency) include oxaliplatin, carboplatin, cyclophosphamide (<1500 mg/m^2), irinotecan, doxorubicin, daunorubicin, epirubicin, idarubicin, ifosfamide, cytarabine (>1 g/m^2), and ixabepilone.[3] Some of the more commonly administered antiemetics in this setting are listed in **Table 1**.

Despite the administration of prophylactic antiemetics to patients receiving high-risk regimens, some patients experience breakthrough nausea and vomiting,[2] which can be severe. Initial evaluation should focus on ensuring that adequate antiemetic therapy was actually administered and ruling out other factors that could be responsible for persistent emesis. Such factors include, but are not limited to, use of opioid analgesics or certain antibiotics (eg, erythromycin), presence of central nervous system (CNS) metastases, or gastrointestinal obstruction, hypercalcemia, or abdominopelvic radiotherapy.[2]

Once it has been concluded that the breakthrough nausea and emesis are due to the chemotherapy and not another concerning process, treatment may focus on supportive measures. The majority of patients who have breakthrough emesis have derived some benefit from the original antiemetic regimen; thus, the original regimens should usually be retained.[2] If not already being taken, corticosteroids, such as dexamethasone, or any of the shorter-acting 5-hydroxytryptamine3 (5-HT3) receptor antagonists (eg, granisetron, ondansetron, or dolasetron) may be prescribed. If the high-therapeutic-index antiemetics are already employed as part of a regimen, then addition of lower-therapeutic-index drugs (**Table 2**) should be considered, including dopaminergic antagonists and benzodiazepines.

Table 1 Commonly administered antiemetics	
Antiemetic Drug	**Dose and Schedule**
High-therapeutic-index drugs	
5-HT3 receptor antagonists	
Granisetron (Kytril)	1 mg PO once daily x 2–3 d
Ondansetron (Zofran)	8 mg PO twice daily x 2–3 d
Dolasetron (Anzemet)	100 mg PO daily x 2–3 d
Corticosteroids	
Dexamethasone (PO)	8 mg PO twice daily starting 24 h after the start of chemotherapy for 4 d (cisplatin) 8 mg PO daily for 2 d (non-cisplatin)
Neurokinin 1 antagonists	
Aprepitant (Emend)	80 mg PO daily for 2 d starting 24 h after the start of chemotherapy

Data from Hesketh P. Chemotherapy-induced nausea and vomiting. N Engl J Med 2008;358: 2482–94.

Table 2	
Low-therapeutic-index antiemetic drugs	
Dopaminergic Antagonists	
Metoclopramide (Reglan)	20 mg or 0.5 mg/kg PO in delayed emesis 4 times daily starting 24 h after the start of chemotherapy for 3–4 d
Prochlorperazine (Compazine)	5–10 mg PO every 6 h as needed
Benzodiazepines	
Lorazepam (Ativan)	1 mg PO every 4–6 h as needed
Others	
Dronabinol	5 mg/m^2 every 2–4 h as needed
Nabilone	1–2 mg twice daily or as needed
Olanzapine	10 mg on days 2–4

Data from Hesketh P. Chemotherapy-induced nausea and vomiting. N Engl J Med 2008;358: 2482–94.

Gastrointestinal Complications

Chemotherapy-induced gastrointestinal toxicity is a common occurrence, can be debilitating and, in some cases life threatening. Such gastrointestinal complications include, but are not limited to, diarrhea, constipation, colitis (neutropenic/typhlitis and C. difficile-induced), and intestinal perforation.[4]

Diarrhea

Diarrhea is a common complication that can be a result of the cancer itself or the chemotherapy. The fluoropyrimidines, especially 5-fluorouracil (5-FU) and capecitabine, as well as the topoisomerase-I inhibitor irinotecan, are the chemotherapy agents most commonly associated with diarrhea.[4] Initial assessment of the patient presenting with chemotherapy-related diarrhea should focus on establishing the severity, which may be assessed using the National Cancer Institute Common Toxicity Criteria (NCI CTC) grading scale (**Table 3**).[5] Patients should also be assessed for complicating factors, such as abdominal cramping, nausea/vomiting, dizziness, significant dehydration, fever, sepsis, neutropenia, overt bleeding, or decreased performance status. Patients with grade 1 to 2 diarrhea and no complicating factors may be initially managed conservatively in the outpatient setting.[1] The mainstays of outpatient treatment for chemotherapy-induced diarrhea are the opiate agonists loperamide (Imodium) and diphenoxylate (Lomotil).[1] Loperamide, the standard dose of which is 4 mg upfront followed by 2 mg every four hours, has been recommended in treatment guidelines.[1] Grade 3 or 4 diarrhea along with any of the above signs or symptoms indicates the need for hospital admission with full diagnostic workup, including standard chemistry screen, complete blood count, and stool culture, as well as aggressive treatment with intravenous (IV) fluids, antibiotics, and consideration of octreotide therapy.

Constipation

Constipation in a patient receiving chemotherapy is relatively common, occurring in up to 33% of patients.[6,7] It may be due to the chemotherapy itself (most typically seen with the vinca alkaloids, vincristine, vinblastine, and vinorelbine[6]), due to poor oral intake, or supportive drugs, such as opioid analgesics or antiemetic drugs that may

Table 3
National Cancer Institute common toxicity criteria for chemotherapy-induced diarrhea

Grade	No Colostomy	Colostomy	BMT
0	None	None	None
1	Increase of <4 stools per day over pretreatment	Mild increase in loose, watery colostomy output compared with pretreatment	>500 mL–1000 mL of diarrhea/day
2	Increase of 4–6 stools per day or nocturnal stools; moderate cramping	Moderate increase in loose, watery colostomy output compared with pretreatment, but not interfering with normal activity	>1000 mL–1500 mL diarrhea/day
3	Increase of 7 or more stools per day; severe cramping, incontinence	Severe increase in loose, watery colostomy output compared with pretreatment, interfering with normal activity	>1500 mL diarrhea/day
4	>10 stools/day; grossly bloody diarrhea, need for parenteral support	Physiologic consequences requiring intensive care or hemodynamic collapse	Severe abdominal pain ± ileus

Abbreviation: BMT, bone marrow transplant.
From Common Toxicity Criteria, version 3.0, National Institutes of Health, National Cancer Institute. Available at: www.ctep.info.nih.gov.

slow intestinal transit time. Therapy includes the laxatives docusate, senna, or bisacodyl. If these agents are not effective, magnesium salts, polyethylene glycol (Miralax), lactulose, or sorbitol are often effective.[8] More invasive measures, such as suppositories, enemas, or manual disimpaction, are contraindicated in neutropenic patients, as these measures may increase the risk for infection.

Colitis

The 3 most common types of colitis that have been described in association with chemotherapy are neutropenic enterocolitis, ischemic colitis, and *Clostridium difficile*-associated colitis. When one of these diagnoses is suspected, abdominal imaging with computed tomography (CT) scan should be obtained, in addition to the routine laboratory evaluation. Empiric antibiotic therapy is also appropriate in this setting.

Intestinal Perforation

Therapy-related intestinal perforation is most commonly seen in patients with metastatic colorectal cancer but may also be seen in patients with any malignancy that involves the gastrointestinal tract. The reported incidence in patients treated for metastatic colorectal cancer is in the range of 1% to 2%.[9,10] A special situation is the increased risk of intestinal perforation in patients treated with the monoclonal antibody bevacizumab (Avastin), which targets cancers expressing vascular endothelial growth factor.

Neutropenia and Infectious Complications

Almost all chemotherapeutic drugs, administered either as single-agent therapy or as part of multidrug regimens, are capable of inducing neutropenia to varying degrees.

The definition of neutropenia varies from institution to institution but is usually defined as an absolute neutrophil count less than 500 cells/μL or less than 1,000 cells/μL with a predicted nadir of less than 500 cells/μL.[8] Isolated neutropenia without signs or symptoms of infection does not require prophylactic antibiotic treatment. However, fever in a neutropenic patient should be considered a medical emergency.[11] Fever in a neutropenic patient is usually defined as a single temperature greater than 38.3°C (101.3°F) or a sustained temperature greater than 38°C (100.4°F) for more than 1 hour.[12]

All febrile neutropenic patients should have a careful history and detailed physical examination, including examination of the skin, mucous membranes, sinuses, fundi, and visual inspection of the perianal area. Even with a detailed physical examination, signs of infection/inflammation are likely to be subtle in the absence of neutrophils. Digital rectal examination (and rectal temperatures) should be avoided, given the increased risk of introducing bacteria into the bloodstream. However, if a perirectal abscess or prostatitis is suspected, gentle rectal examination can be performed after broad-spectrum antibiotics have been administered. All indwelling or recent line sites should be carefully examined. Not all infected neutropenic patients will present with a fever, especially the elderly and patients receiving corticosteroids.[11] Signs of sepsis other than fever, such as hypotension or cardiopulmonary compromise, may be the only initial signs of occult infection.

Initial laboratory evaluation should include complete blood count with differential, complete chemistry panel with liver function tests and lipase and a full set of cultures, including sputum, urine and blood drawn both peripherally and from all indwelling lines. Imaging with chest radiographs should be obtained even if the patient does not have pulmonary symptoms. Chest x-ray findings are often minimal or absent even in patients with pneumonia. Chest axial CT scanning may demonstrate abnormalities such as pneumonia even when the chest x-ray is normal.[10]

If localizing signs or symptoms are present, consider additional imaging of the CNS, sinuses, abdomen, or pelvis or obtaining additional laboratory tests, such as stool studies or direct fluorescent antibody testing for herpes simplex virus (HSV) or varicella zoster virus (VZV). Lumbar puncture is not performed routinely but should be performed in patients who have a change in mental status and/or CNS signs or symptoms.

Empiric antibiotics should be initiated promptly in all febrile neutropenic patients.[12] Early studies documented up to 70% mortality if initiation of antibiotics was delayed even more than a few hours.[13] Numerous antibiotic regimens have been studied as initial empiric therapy, some as monotherapy and others as part of 2-drug combination regimens. None has been shown to be clearly superior,[14–17] and currently, there is no clear optimal choice for empiric therapy. Currently recommended regimens for empiric treatment of febrile neutropenia are aimed against gram-negative bacilli, especially *Pseudomonas aeruginosa*. Empiric gram-positive antibiotics have not been found to have significant clinical benefit.[18,19] A meta-analysis of 7 randomized, controlled trials failed to demonstrate a reduction in all-cause mortality when empiric gram-positive antibiotic coverage was added to standard empiric therapy in patients with febrile neutropenia.[20] However, vancomycin should be added to the empiric regimen in patients presenting with cardiovascular compromise, suspected entry of bacteria through cutaneous portals (eg, mucositis, skin, or catheter sites), a history of methicillin-resistant *Staphylococcus aureus* (MRSA) colonization, or having received recent antibiotic prophylaxis.[21] Upfront empiric anaerobic or antifungal therapy for initial presentation with febrile neutropenia is not currently recommended. Specific anaerobic coverage should be added if there is evidence of necrotizing mucositis, sinusitis, periodontal abscess, perirectal abscess/cellulitis, intra-abdominal or pelvic infection, typhlitis (necrotizing neutropenic colitis), or anaerobic bacteremia. Recommendations for initial empiric antibiotic use, adapted from the Infectious Disease Society of America Guidelines 2002, appear in **Table 4**.[12] These guidelines are scheduled to be updated and revised in 2009.

With regard to the use of colony-stimulating factors (CSFs) (eg, filgrastim, a.k.a. granulocyte-CSF) in febrile neutropenic patients, one meta-analysis[22] did show a reduction in duration of neutropenia and length of hospitalization. However, there was no overall decrease in mortality; thus, CSFs are not routinely administered to patients with fever and neutropenia. Special circumstances in which the use of CSFs may be considered include critically ill patients, such as those with pneumonia, hypotension, or organ dysfunction, and patients whose bone marrow recovery is expected to be especially prolonged.[11]

Recently, several randomized trials have examined the feasibility of outpatient management of patients with low-risk febrile neutropenia.[23,24] However, ensuring that truly low-risk patients are selected is problematic, and, as a result, the outpatient strategy should not be viewed as the current standard of care for febrile neutropenic patients.

Therapy-Induced Anemia and Fatigue

Fatigue is a common problem for patients who are undergoing cancer treatment, although it is consistently underreported to health care providers.[25] Fatigue secondary to malignancy is highly subjective, often described as persistent tiredness, despite adequate rest, that limits one's daily routine.[26] Chemotherapy may contribute directly or indirectly to the development of fatigue,[27] with anemia being the most common reversible cause of fatigue in this patient population.

Anemia is a common complication in patients receiving myelosuppressive chemotherapy. The vast majority of patients receiving such therapy develop anemia of mild-moderate severity.[28] The initial approach to the anemic patient receiving chemotherapy should rule out blood loss from other sources, including hemolysis, and

Table 4
2002 Infectious Disease Society of America guidelines for the use of antimicrobial agents in neutropenic patients with cancer
Initial Antibiotic Therapy
Monotherapy: Cefepime or ceftazidime or imipenem or meropenem
Dual therapy: Aminoglycoside plus anti-pseudomonal beta-lactam, cephalosporin (cefepime or ceftazidime), or carbapenem   Vancomycin should be added to either monotherapy or dual therapy only if criteria are met[a]   Oral therapy (only for low-risk adults):   Ciprofloxacin plus amoxicillin-clavulanate

[a] Vancomycin should be added for hypotension or other signs of cardiovascular compromise, clinically serious suspected intravascular catheter-related infection, colonization with MRSA or penicillin/cephalosporin-resistant pneumococci, mucositis, history of positive blood cultures for gram-positive cocci, and for patients with recent quinolone prophylaxis.

Data from Hughes WT, Armstrong D, Bodey GP, et al. 2002 guidelines for the use of antimicrobial agents in neutropenic patients with cancer. Clin Infect Dis 2002;34:730.

subsequently assess for deficiencies of iron, folate and vitamin B12. Management of symptomatic anemia from chemotherapy-induced myelosuppression includes transfusion of packed red blood cells and/or the administration of the erythropoiesis-stimulating agents, erythropoietin or darbepoietin. Symptomatic improvements following transfusion occur almost immediately, while clinical responses to the erythropoiesis-stimulating agents are more prolonged, often a matter of weeks.[29] In these circumstances, transfusion may be particularly appropriate in severely symptomatic patients. Current guidelines recommend that erythropoiesis-stimulating agents be administered only to patients with nonhematologic malignancies who have symptomatic anemia (hemoglobin <10 g/dL) that is directly related to ongoing treatment with myelosuppressive chemotherapy.[29] The erythropoiesis-stimulating agents have been associated with an increased incidence of cardiovascular and thromboembolic events as well as decreased survival when administered to patients whose anemia is not due to concomitant use of chemotherapy.[30]

Fatigue may also be secondary to inadequate nutrition secondary to a myriad of chemotherapy-induced gastrointestinal side effects, such as anorexia, nausea, vomiting, mucositis, odynophagia, dysphagia, constipation, abdominal pain, distention, and/or obstruction. Patients with poor dietary intake or decreased absorption may need inpatient supplemental nutrition as well as further assessment by a nutritionist. In the immediate setting, interventions should focus on reducing or eliminating chemotherapy-related side effects such as nausea, vomiting, or diarrhea, all of which prevent adequate nutrition.

Laboratory evaluation of the cancer patient with significant fatigue should include full chemistry panel with calcium, magnesium, and phosphorous, full panel of liver function tests, lactate dehydrogenase, thyroid-stimulating hormone and a complete blood count with differential. All electrolyte imbalances (particularly sodium, potassium, calcium, phosphorus, and magnesium) should be corrected with appropriate supplementation.

Chemotherapy-Induced Liver Toxicity

Chemotherapy agents may lead to a wide spectrum of hepatotoxicity, ranging from clinically asymptomatic transaminitis to severe acute hepatitis, or occasionally vascular complications such as hepatic venoocclusive disease (VOD).[31] The etiology of liver dysfunction in the patient receiving chemotherapy may not be immediately apparent. Besides chemotherapy, other etiologies include enlarging hepatic tumor burden, pre-existing hepatic disease, and hepatotoxic effects of other drugs.[32,33] Signs suggestive of chemotherapy-induced toxicity include lack of pre-existing liver disease and onset of hepatic insufficiency in proximity to the time of chemotherapy administration. Chemotherapy-induced liver toxicity may be mediated either through direct toxic effects or worsening of pre-existing liver disease (eg, viral hepatitis).

Patients with pre-existing liver disease, such as hepatitis B (HBV) or C (HCV), who are receiving cytotoxic chemotherapy are susceptible to exacerbation of their underlying liver disease and are at increased risk for chemotherapy-induced hepatotoxicity. For patients with known HBV, there is an increased incidence of reactivation in those receiving systemic chemotherapy.[34] Although multiple studies have shown increased incidence of grade 1 (mild) and 2 (moderate) transaminitis in patients with anti-HCV antibodies treated with various chemotherapeutic regimens, severe transaminitis is uncommon.[35] However, positive HCV serology does increase the risk for hepatic VOD in patients undergoing high-dose chemotherapy and hematopoietic stem cell transplantation (HSCT).

Chemotherapy-Associated Renal Toxicity

Almost all chemotherapy agents are capable of causing at least some degree of renal insufficiency, either directly or indirectly (eg, dehydration secondary to nausea and vomiting). Manifestations of such therapy-related nephrotoxicity may range from asymptomatic elevation of serum creatinine to acute renal failure requiring dialysis.

Table 5 provides a limited list of specific chemotherapeutic agents and their associated manifestations of renal toxicity. Non–chemotherapy-related renal failure is discussed elsewhere in this issue.

Chemotherapy-Induced Cardiotoxicity

Many chemotherapeutic agents have been associated with cardiotoxicity and place the cancer patient at an increased risk for cardiovascular complications. This risk rises if there is pre-existing heart disease.[36] Chemotherapy-related cardiovascular complications may occur several days to weeks following administration or even years following exposure. Anthracyclines, such as doxorubicin, daunorubicin, and epirubicin, are most frequently associated with causing cardiotoxicity[48] and typically cause a symptomatic dilated cardiomyopathy. The patient typically presents with signs and symptoms of new and/or worsening heart failure.

The IV antimetabolite 5-FU is a component of multiple different chemotherapy regimens and, similar to the anthracyclines, is a common cause of chemotherapy-induced cardiotoxicity.[48] This agent most commonly causes chest pain secondary to coronary artery vasospasm.[49] Similar cardiotoxicity is seen with the oral fluoropyrimidine capecitabine (metabolized to 5-FU). Symptomatic patients require hospital admission and possible coronary evaluation with stress testing or angiography.

Table 5
Chemotherapeutic agents associated with renal toxicity

Chemotherapeutic Agent	Nephrotoxic Manifestations
Cisplatin	Hypomagnesemia RTA ARF[37,38]
Cyclophosphamide	Hyponatremia[39] Hemorrhagic cystitis
Ifosfamide	Type 1 (distal) or type II (proximal) RTA[40]
Mitomycin	ARF associated with TTP-HUS[41]
Rituximab	ARF secondary to tumor lysis syndrome[42]
Bevacizumab/sunitinib/sorafenib	Proteinuria/nephrotic syndrome[43]
Cetuximab/panitumumab	Hypomagnesemia[44]
Interleukin-2	Capillary leak syndrome, edema ARF[45,46]
Interferon-alpha	Proteinuria Minimal change nephropathy[47]
Interferon-gamma	Acute tubular necrosis[47]

Abbreviations: ARF, acute renal failure; ATN, acute tubular necrosis; RTA, renal tubular acidosis; TTP-HUS, thrombotic thrombocytopenic purpura–hemolytic uremic syndrome.
Data from Merchan J. Chemotherapy and renal insufficiency. In: Basow DS, editor. UpToDate: Waltham (MA); 2009. Available at: www.uptodate.com.

Trastuzumab (Herceptin) is a monoclonal antibody administered as part of the treatment for breast cancer overexpressing HER2/neu (ErbB2). Trastuzumab-related cardiotoxicity involves a predominantly asymptomatic cardiomyopathy, with an incidence ranging from 7.4% to 17.3% of patients.[50] A decreased left-ventricular ejection fraction (LVEF) is noted only by routine screening with transthoracic echocardiogram and is not typically manifested by report of symptoms. Much less commonly, trastuzumab is associated with symptomatic heart failure, occurring in 0.6% to 4.1% of patients.[50]

Sunitinib is a nonspecific, small molecule, tyrosine kinase inhibitor and is used for the treatment of renal cell carcinoma and refractory gastrointestinal stromal tumors. Sunitinib-related cardiovascular toxicity includes hypertension at a frequency ranging from 15% to 47%,[49] symptomatic heart failure (approx 8%),[49] and an asymptomatic decrease in LVEF in 10% to 28% of patients.[51]

At this time, it is unclear as to whether patients with left-ventricular dysfunction secondary to chemotherapy benefit from typical heart failure medical therapy, specifically angiotensin-converting enzyme (ACE) inhibitors and beta blockers. Although the data are limited, current evidence suggests clinical benefit with ACE inhibitors as first-line therapy for both asymptomatic left-ventricular dysfunction and overt heart failure due to systolic dysfunction.[52]

Neurologic Complications of Cancer Chemotherapy

Neurologic toxicities associated with antineoplastic drug treatment may range from headaches and cranial or other neuropathies to aseptic meningitis, transverse myelopathy, visual loss, seizures, vasculopathies, cerebrovascular accident, acute encephalopathy, acute cerebellar syndrome, and dementia.[53–55]

One of the more common chemotherapy-induced neurotoxicities is the sensory neuropathy seen with the taxanes, paclitaxel (Taxol) and docetaxel (Taxotere),[56] and the vinca alkaloids (eg, vincristine).[57] Sensory neuropathy is usually manifested by paresthesias of the fingertips, palms of the hands, and soles of the feet. Docetaxel has also been associated with the development of Lhermitte's sign, an electric shock-like sensation radiating down the spine upon neck flexion.[58] Vincristine may, in some patients, be associated with various cranial neuropathies (usually oculomotor) or motor neuropathies, often with profound weakness, bilateral foot drop, and/or wrist drop.

Methotrexate has been associated with a wide range of neurotoxicity, including aseptic meningitis, transverse myelopathy, acute and subacute encephalopathy, and leukoencephalopathy.[59] Both aseptic meningitis as well as transverse myelopathy (isolated spinal cord dysfunction) may be seen following intrathecal administration of methotrexate;[60] however, the incidence of aseptic meningitis in this setting is much higher than that for myelopathy.[60] Acute encephalopathy, presenting with somnolence, confusion, and/or seizures within 24 hours of treatment, is most frequently seen after high-dose methotrexate.[60] Subacute encephalopathy, characterized by transient focal neurologic deficits, confusion, and occasionally seizures, may occur approximately 6 days after methotrexate administration.[61] Leukoencephalopathy, with characteristic cognitive impairment, is the major delayed complication of methotrexate occurring months to years following treatment.[60]

Overdosage with intrathecal methotrexate may result in seizures, acute myelopathy, encephalopathy, coma, severe cardiopulmonary compromise, and death.[62] Emergent therapy consists of intrathecal glucarpidase (carboxypeptidase G2), ventriculolumbar perfusion/cerebrospinal fluid exchange, IV folinic acid (Leucovorin), and alkaline diuresis.[63,64]

Oral Complications and Mucositis

Mucositis is the most frequently encountered oral complication of systemic chemotherapy, affecting approximately 35% to 40% of patients.[65–67] The frequency is even higher in patients undergoing HSCT. Xerostomia as a consequence of systemic cytotoxic chemotherapy is much less common. Grading of mucositis severity is according to the NCI CTC, as described in **Table 6**.[68]

The cytotoxic drugs most commonly associated with mucositis are cytarabine, doxorubicin, etoposide, 5-FU, and methotrexate.[69,70] Severe erosive mucositis often shows as multiple shallow ulcerations with a pseudomembranous appearance, which coalesce to form large painful lesions. Sequelae may include severe pain, impaired oral intake with poor nutrition, spontaneous bleeding if thrombocytopenic, and even secondary infection and sepsis, especially if there is concurrent neutropenia. The majority of oral infections secondary to mucositis are caused by *Candida albicans*,[71] with the remaining cases predominantly due to HSV.[72] Localized therapy for oropharyngeal candidiasis consists of clotrimazole or nystatin, whereas systemic antifungal treatment is typically administered with oral fluconazole. Empiric antiviral therapy with acyclovir or valacyclovir is appropriate.[72] The presence of such severe mucositis would necessitate hospital admission for pain control with opiates, usually morphine,[73] and administration of parenteral nutrition.

Treatment of less severe mucositis is supportive and typically includes proper oral hygiene as well as mucosal protectants and topical analgesia. Topical lidocaine solutions provide pain relief and are frequently combined with coating agents. One such mixture of viscous lidocaine, sodium bicarbonate, and diphenhydramine is commonly referred to as "miracle mouthwash."

Hypersensitivity Reactions to Systemic Chemotherapy

The vast majority of hypersensitivity reactions induced by chemotherapy are type I, immunoglobulin E-mediated, allergic reactions, occurring in a range from 30 minutes to 72 hours postinfusion. Common symptoms include flushing, pruritus, nausea, angioedema, bronchospasm, laryngospasm, dyspnea, wheezing, alterations in heart rate and blood pressure, back pain, fever, and all types of rashes/urticaria. High rates of hypersensitivity reactions have been described with platinum-based agents (carboplatin, oxaliplatin), L-asparaginase, taxanes (paclitaxel, docetaxel), epidophyllotoxins

Table 6		
The national cancer institute common toxicity criteria grading of the severity of mucositis		
Grade	**Clinical Examination**	**Functional or Symptomatic**
1	Erythema of the mucosa	Minimal symptoms, normal diet
2	Patchy ulcerations or pseudomembranes	Symptomatic but can eat and swallow modified diet
3	Confluent ulcerations or pseudomembranes; bleeding with minor trauma	Symptomatic and unable to adequately aliment or hydrate orally
4	Tissue necrosis; significant spontaneous bleeding; life-threatening consequences	Symptoms associated with life-threatening consequences
5	Death	Death

Data from Cancer Therapy Evaluation Program. Common terminology criteria for adverse events, version 3.0. Available at: http://ctep.cancer.gov/protocolDevelopment/electronic_applications/docs/ctcaev3.pdf.

(etoposide, teniposide), procarbazine, and recombinant monoclonal antibodies (rituximab, trastuzumab, alemtuzumab, cetuximab).[74,75] Premedication with a corticosteroid reduces, but does not eliminate, the risk of hypersensitivity reactions. Treatment depends on the severity of the reaction (**Box 1**)[76] but always includes the immediate discontinuation of the offending agent and close monitoring of the patient.

Bleomycin has been associated with 2 distinct hypersensitivity reactions. This drug may induce an acute hypersensitivity pneumonitis, presenting as dyspnea, cough, and rash.[77] Bleomycin-induced hypersensitivity has similar radiographic findings as those in the more common interstitial pneumonitis; however, hypersensitivity pneumonitis is uniquely associated with peripheral eosinophilia. Corticosteroid therapy has been shown to facilitate resolution of symptoms.[78] In contrast, bleomycin infusions may also be accompanied by a febrile anaphylactoid reaction known as the hyperpyrexia syndrome, occurring in approximately 1% of patients, particularly those with lymphoma.[75] High fever is followed by excessive sweating, which may be accompanied by wheezing, mental confusion, and low urine output and hypotension.[75] Onset may be immediate or occur up to days following the dose.[78] Treatment is supportive with IV hydration, steroid therapy, and H1-receptor antagonists.[78] Rarely, this condition may progress to fulminant hyperpyrexia with disseminated intravascular coagulation.[78]

Extravasation Injury

Cytotoxic chemotherapeutic agents are classified as irritants or vesicants based on their likelihood of causing local toxicity.[79] Irritant and vesicant classifications represent the ends of a spectrum and are not absolute; the extent of tissue injury often depends on the amount of drug that has extravasated.

Irritant drugs cause a localized inflammatory reaction. Examination may reveal warmth, erythema, and tenderness in the area; however there should be no signs of tissue necrosis.[79] There are no long-lasting sequelae following extravasation of irritant drugs.

Vesicant chemotherapeutic drugs are likely to cause tissue necrosis with more severe and widespread tissue injury. The most commonly used vesicant chemotherapeutic agents are the anthracyclines. Initial physical signs may include only localized burning with mild swelling; subsequently, approximately 48 to 72 hours following

---

Box 1
Recommendations for treatment of hypersensitivity reactions in patients receiving chemotherapy

Discontinue drug immediately

For severe reactions with bronchospasm or hypotension, administer epinephrine 0.35 to 0.50 mL of a 1:1000 solution intramuscularly every 15 to 20 minutes or until the reaction subsides or a total of 6 doses

Administer diphenhydramine 50 mg IV

If hypotension is present that does not respond to epinephrine, administer IV fluids

If wheezing is present that does not respond to epinephrine, administer 0.35 mL of nebulized albuterol solution

Administer parenteral corticosteroids (eg, methylprednisolone 125 mg, hydrocortisone 100 mg, dexamethasone 8 mg). Although corticosteroids have no effect on the initial reaction, they can block late allergic symptoms

Data from Albanell J, Baselga J. Systemic therapy emergencies. Semin Oncol 2000;27:347.

extravasation of drug, there may be worsening pain, redness, skin desquamation, and/or blistering.[80] In the next several weeks, more typical signs of necrosis may be present, including eschar formation with ulceration.[79]

Local application of ice or cold packs, with concurrent vasoconstriction and limitation of drug spread, is appropriate for all extravasation injuries except those caused by the vinca alkaloids (vincristine, vinblastine, vinorelbine) and epipodophyllotoxins such as etoposide.[81] In the case of the latter, heat is recommended,[82] facilitating drug removal via the increased blood flow through the affected area.

Nonhealing ulcers caused by vesicant drug extravasation may require surgical consultation, debridement, and skin grafting.[79] Failure of initial conservative management with signs of persistent erythema, swelling, worsening pain, or the presence of large areas of tissue necrosis and/or skin ulceration are indications for surgery.[83] If left untreated, adverse sequelae, such as nerve compression syndromes, permanent joint stiffness, contractures, and neurologic dysfunction, may occur.[84] Specific antidotes for particular chemotherapeutic agents have been suggested to prevent necrosis and ulceration following extravasation. These include sodium thiosulfate for mechlorethamine/nitrogen mustard extravasations, topical application or subcutaneous injection of dimethylsulfoxide for anthracycline or mitomycin extravasations, local injection of hyaluronidase for the vinca alkaloids, paclitaxel, epipodophyllotoxins, and ifosfamide, and systemic administration of dexrazoxane for anthracycline extravasations.[79] Unfortunately, no randomized trials have been performed to support any of these interventions, and thus, there is no consensus on the proper use of these agents.[77]

HEMATOPOIETIC STEM CELL TRANSPLANT–RELATED INFECTIOUS COMPLICATIONS

HSCT refers to transplantation of hematopoietic stem cells obtained from bone marrow, peripheral blood, or cord blood. Hematopoietic stem cells obtained from the patient him- or herself are referred to as autologous, and hematopoietic stem cells obtained from someone other than the patient are referred to as allogeneic. Complications seen in the post-transplant period can be roughly divided into infectious and noninfectious categories.

Infectious Complications in HSCT

The likely causative agent of an infectious complication following HSCT is related to the timing post-transplant and may be influenced by additional factors, such as the duration and severity of neutropenia, as well as the presence of immunosuppressive medications. The post-transplant period is divided into the following designations: (1) Pre-engraftment period: less than 30 days after HSCT, (2) Immediate postengraftment period: 30 to 100 days post-HSCT, and (3) Late postengraftment: more than 100 days post-HSCT.

Infections in the Pre-Engraftment Period

The infectious complications seen during this early period do not significantly differ between autologous and allogeneic transplants. The major risk factors for infection during this period include mucocutaneous damage (eg, mucositis) and neutropenia.[85] Aerobic gram-positive and gram-negative bacteria account for most documented infections during this granulocytopenic period.[86] Gram-positive bacteria include coagulase-negative Staphylococci, *Staphylococcus aureus*, viridans streptococci, and others. Gram-negative infections may be caused by Legionella spp., *Pseudomonas aeruginosa*, Enterobacteriaceae, and *Stenotrophomonas maltophilia*, and other bacteria.[87] The most common sites of bacterial infection include intravascular devices and the bloodstream, lungs, and gastrointestinal tract.

The likelihood of fungal infections during the pre-engraftment period is positively correlated with the severity and duration of neutropenia. The vast majority of patients are now treated with prophylactic fluconazole during this period, which has significantly reduced, but not eliminated, the occurrence of invasive candidiasis. When present, candidal infections may be localized (such as to the oral, esophageal, or genital area) or disseminated.[88] Skin lesions, usually erythematous and maculopapular in nature, can be the first evidence of disseminated candidiasis. The incidence of infection with triazole-resistant Candida species, such as *C. krusei and C. glabrata*, has increased, likely as a result of prophylactic therapy.[89] Infections caused by molds (eg, Aspergillus), may also occur during this phase,[88] usually after 10 to 14 days of neutropenia. The risk for infection from molds is higher in the allogeneic group than in the autologous group. The major clinical manifestation of infection with these molds is pulmonary infection. Involvement of the sinuses, CNS, and skin may also occur.

The major viruses encountered during the pre-engraftment period are HSV and the respiratory viruses. The majority of HSV infections in HSCT recipients occur as reactivation of latent HSV-1 infection,[85] the rate of which is approximately 70% and appears comparable after either autologous or allogeneic transplantation.[87] Clinically, HSV reactivations typically present with severe mucositis, but patients may also complain of symptoms of esophagitis. Reactivation of HSV-2 infection in the genital or perineal area accounts for only 10% to 15% of all HSV infections in HSCT patients.[90] Prophylaxis with acyclovir or valacyclovir has markedly reduced the incidence of all herpetic reactivations in this patient population.

The most common respiratory viruses include respiratory syncytial virus (RSV), the parainfluenza viruses, rhinoviruses, and influenza A and B. These infections are seen both in allogeneic and autologous recipients.[91] Initial clinical manifestations typically include upper respiratory tract symptoms (eg, rhinorrhea, sinus congestion, sore throat, and otitis media), which almost always precede lower respiratory tract infection (tracheobronchitis, pneumonia).[92] Infection with RSV occurs in more than 50% of HSCT recipients but, usually, is not a severe illness.[93] During community outbreaks, influenza, especially type A, and parainfluenza viruses have been reported as a frequent cause of severe and fatal pneumonia in HSCT recipients.[94]

Infections in the Immediate Postengraftment Period

There is a significant increased risk for infection among recipients of allogeneic transplant in this time period compared with that among those of autologous transplant.[91] Similar to the pre-engraftment stage, mucocutaneous damage increases the risk of infection in both groups; however, additional risk factors for allogeneic transplant recipients include presence of acute graft-versus-host disease (GVHD), impaired cellular immunity, and cytomegalovirus (CMV) reactivation.[91]

Among recipients of autologous transplants, infections occurring between days 30 and 100 post-transplant are most commonly bacterial indwelling catheter infections or viral infections with either VZV reactivation or community respiratory viruses.[91] For allogeneic transplant recipients in the immediate postengraftment period, typical bacterial infections include gram-positive (eg, coagulase-negative staphylococci), catheter-related infections or gram-negative bacteremia, typically with enteric organisms (eg, *Escherichia coli, Klebsiella, Enterobacter*) or *Pseudomonas*, the risk of which is increased in the setting of acute GVHD.[91]

GVHD is also a risk factor for fungal infection (typically Aspergillus), as is concomitant steroid usage and active CMV disease. The incidence of invasive aspergillosis among allogeneic HSCT recipients is 5% to 30%, and the median time of onset of aspergillosis is 6 to 12 weeks after transplantation.[95]

CMV reactivation is very common among allogeneic transplant recipients who are known to be serologically positive for CMV or whose donor was known to be serologically positive for CMV. The incidence is approximately 70% in this population, and such infections most commonly present as fever of unknown origin, interstitial pneumonitis, or enteritis; less often, these patients can develop retinitis, encephalitis, hepatitis, or bone marrow suppression.[95,96] Human herpes virus-6 (HHV-6) reactivation has also been documented in 40% to 60% of HSCT recipients.[97,98] Although most patients are clinically asymptomatic, there are a myriad possible clinical syndromes associated with HHV-6 reactivation, including rash, fever, interstitial pneumonitis,[98] encephalitis,[98] and bone marrow suppression.[98] Infection with respiratory viruses, such as RSV, influenza and parainfluenza, and rhinovirus, continues to occur during the immediate postengraftment period. Reactivation of adenovirus infection occurs in greater than 80% of autologous and allogeneic HSCT recipients but causes severe disease in very few patients.[99]

Infections in the Late Postengraftment Period

Infections during this period are typically seen only in recipients of allogeneic transplants. Risk for infectious complications is increased in the setting of chronic GVHD (with resultant functional hyposplenism, cellular and humoral immune dysfunction) and prolonged steroid use.[91]

Typical bacterial pathogens during this time period include the encapsulated organisms (*Streptococcus pneumoniae, Hemophilus influenzae, Neisseria meningitidis*),[100] staphylococci, and gram-negative bacteria (eg, *Pseudomonas*).[101] Fungal infections are uncommon beyond 100 days post-transplant, except in the patient receiving chronic on-going immunosuppressive medications.

Common viral agents in the late postengraftment period include CMV and the respiratory viruses (as in the early postengraftment time) with the addition of VZV reactivation.[91] The incidence of VZV reactivation is approximately equal among allogeneic and autologous HSCT recipients (20%–40%); however, it is more common among children (up to 90% by year 1) compared with adults.[102] VZV reactivation most commonly presents with cutaneous rash or postherpetic neuralgia.

Noninfectious Complications of HSCT

Graft-versus-host disease

Acute GVHD is defined as occurring within the first 100 days following allogeneic HSCT, with established neutrophil engraftment. GVHD is not seen following autologous HSCT. The incidence varies widely among recipients of allogeneic HSCT, from 20% to 80%; however, it is most common among recipients of an HLA-identical matched unrelated transplant. The skin, liver, gastrointestinal tract, and the hematopoietic system are the principal target organs in patients with acute GVHD.[103]

Typically, the initial (and most common) sign of acute GVHD is a maculopapular rash, usually involving the neck, ears, shoulders, the palms of the hands, and the soles of the feet.[103] Following skin involvement, the liver and gastrointestinal tract are the second most commonly involved organs in acute GVHD.[91] Liver damage from GVHD involves the small bile ducts, leading to cholestasis. Hepatic involvement is manifested by abnormal liver function tests, with the earliest and most common finding being a rise in the serum conjugated bilirubin and alkaline phosphatase. It is important to remember that these laboratory values are nonspecific, and a full differential diagnosis, including possible hepatic VOD, viral hepatitis, and drug toxicity (eg, cyclosporine A), needs to be considered. Acute GVHD of the gastrointestinal tract is characterized by diarrhea and abdominal cramping. The severity of gastrointestinal involvement is determined by the volume of diarrhea, which in extreme cases can exceed 10 L/d. The diarrhea may initially be watery but frequently becomes bloody, resulting in significant transfusion requirements.[104] Maintenance of adequate fluid balance may be extremely difficult in such patients. Notably, diarrhea is a common occurrence following HSCT and may be due not only to acute GVHD but also may be secondary to infection (eg, CMV, *C. difficile* toxin-induced) or the preparative chemotherapy regimen.

The diagnosis of acute GVHD can be readily made on clinical grounds alone in the patient who presents with a classic rash, abdominal cramps with diarrhea, and a rising serum bilirubin concentration within the first 100 days following transplantation.[103] Histologic confirmation via biopsy is often required to confirm a diagnosis of acute GVHD.

The severity of GVHD is assessed based on the extent of involvement of the skin, liver, and gastrointestinal tract (**Table 7**). This is subsequently combined to produce an overall grade,[103] which has both therapeutic and prognostic implications. **Table 7** shows the staging of acute GVHD.

First-line therapy of acute GVHD is administration of corticosteroids. For limited skin GVHD (stage 1–2), low-dose prednisone, 1 mg/kg/d orally, may be administered. In addition, topical corticosteroids may be useful: 1% triamcinolone twice daily for any facial rash and 0.1% triamcinolone twice daily for truncal skin involvement.[91] For any stage 3 to 4 skin GVHD or any liver/gastrointestinal tract involvement, first-line therapy is high-dose methylprednisolone, 62.5 mg/m^2 per dose IV given twice daily.[91]

Chronic GVHD occurs after 100 days from allogeneic HSCT. The majority of patients who develop chronic GVHD will have experienced some signs of prior acute GVHD.[91] The chronic form of this complication may develop immediately following the acute GVHD period (first 100 days), or it may follow a quiescent period during which the acute GVHD briefly resolved.[91] Similar to acute GVHD, the chronic form most commonly involves the skin. However, unlike acute GVHD, the presenting organ involvement may be more highly variable, with involvement not only of the liver and gastrointestinal tract but also of the mouth, eyes, lungs, and joints. Symptoms often resemble those associated with autoimmune disorders, such as lichenoid skin changes, sicca syndrome, chronic hepatitis, and bronchiolitis obliterans.[91] Risk factors associated with decreased survival in patients with chronic GVHD include extensive skin involvement (>50% of the BSA), thrombocytopenia (<100,000 platelets/µL), and an onset immediately following acute GVHD.[91] First-line, recommended therapy for chronic GVHD includes the corticosteroid prednisone with or without cyclosporine A. Current recommendations include initiating antimicrobial prophylaxis

Table 7			
Staging of acute graft-versus-host disease			
Stage	**Skin Rash**	**Liver/Total Bilirubin**	**GI Tract/Volume of Diarrhea**
1	<25% involvement	2.0–3.0 mg/dL	>500 mL/day
2	25%–50% involved	3.1–6.0 mg/dL	>1000 mL/day
3	Generalized erythroderma	6.1–15 mg/dL	>1500 mL/day
4	Bullae	>15 mg/dL	Severe abdominal pain, bleeding, ileus

Data from Couriel D, Caldera H, Champlin R, et al. Acute graft-versus-host disease: pathophysiology, clinical manifestations, and management. Cancer 2004;101:1936.

at the time of diagnosis or start of immunosuppressive medications. First-line thera-pies include penicillin V and acyclovir for antibacterial and antiviral prophylaxis, respectively. Prophylactic treatment for Pneumocystis carinii infection with double-strength sulfamethoxazole-trimethoprim (Bactrim, Cotrimaxazole) should also be considered.[91]

Hepatic Venoocclusive Disease/Sinusoidal Obstruction Syndrome

Hepatic VOD, also known as hepatic sinusoidal obstruction syndrome, is induced by damage to the hepatic endothelial cell as well as the hepatocyte. It is characterized by sudden weight gain, peripheral edema, new-onset ascites, hepatomegaly, right upper quadrant pain, and jaundice;[105] occurrence is most often within the first 6 weeks following hematopoietic cell transplantation.[106] Risk factors include use of pretrans-plant conditioning regimens containing busulfan, unrelated donor transplant, pre-ex-isting liver disease or prior radiation to the liver, and peritransplant administration of acyclovir, amphotericin, or methotrexate.[91] The incidence of hepatic VOD after HSCT varies from 5% to 50%.[105] The diagnosis is usually based on clinical presenta-tion with hepatomegaly, weight gain, and jaundice within 20 days of HSCT. Laboratory evaluation may reveal transaminitis and conjugated hyperbilirubinemia. Ultrasound with Doppler evaluation may reveal attenuation or reversal of venous flow or portal venous thrombosis. Patients with severe disease, as evidenced by signs of liver failure (eg, coagulopathy) often develop confusion, bleeding, and renal and cardiopulmonary failure.[104] Treatment in the acute setting is primarily supportive, as approximately 70% of patients will recover spontaneously.[91]

SUMMARY

Chemotherapy and HSCT are associated with a wide array of toxicities and complica-tions, many of which may be encountered in the outpatient setting. An understanding of the organ-specific complications of various chemotherapeutic agents, as well as the infections and GVHD manifestations in the post-transplant period, is critical to successfully treat this patient population.

REFERENCES

1. Kris MG, Gralla RJ, Tyson LB, et al. Controlling delayed vomiting: double-blind, randomized trial comparing placebo, dexamethasone alone, and metoclopra-mide plus dexamethasone in patients receiving cisplatin. J Clin Oncol 1989; 7(1):108–14.
2. Hesketh P. Prevention and treatment chemotherapy-induced nausea and vomiting. Available at: www.uptodate.com. Accessed June 15, 2008.
3. Hesketh P. Chemotherapy-induced nausea and vomiting. N Engl J Med 2008; 358:2482–94.
4. Halmos B, Krishnamurthi S. Enterotoxicity of chemotherapeutic agents. Available at: www.uptodate.com. Accessed June 15, 2008.
5. Common toxicity criteria, version 3.0, National Institutes of Health, National Cancer Institute. Available at: www.ctep.info.nih.gov. Accessed July 15, 2008.
6. Holland JF, Scharlau C, Gailani S, et al. Vincristine treatment of advanced cancer: a cooperative study of 392 cases. Cancer Res 1973;33:1258–64.
7. Anderson H, Scarffe JH, Lambert M, et al. VAD chemotherapy–toxicity and effi-cacy–in patients with multiple myeloma and other lymphoid malignancies. Hematol Oncol 1987;5:213–22.

8. Weed HG. Lactulose vs sorbitol for treatment of obstipation in hospice programs. Mayo Clin Proc 2000;75(5):541.

9. Hurwitz H, Fehrenbacher L, Novotny W, et al. Bevacizumab plus irinotecan, fluorouracil, and leucovorin for metastatic colorectal cancer. N Engl J Med 2004;350: 2335–42.

10. Wright JD, Hagemann A, Rader JS, et al. Bevacizumab combination therapy in recurrent, platinum-refractory, epithelial ovarian carcinoma: a retrospective analysis. Cancer 2006;107:83–9.

11. Robbins G. Fever in the neutropenic adult patient with cancer. Available at: www. uptodate.com. Accessed June 15, 2008.

12. Hughes WT, Armstrong D, Bodey GP, et al. 2002 guidelines for the use of antimicrobial agents in neutropenic patients with cancer. Clin Infect Dis 2002;34(6): 730–51.

13. Schimpff SC, Satterlee W, Young VM, et al. Empiric therapy with carbenicillin and gentamicin for febrile patients with cancer and granulocytopenia. N Engl J Med 1971;284:1061–5.

14. Peacock JE, Herrington DA, Wade JC, et al. Ciprofloxacin plus piperacillin compared with tobramycin plus piperacillin as empirical therapy in febrile neutropenic patients. A randomized, double-blind trial. Ann Intern Med 2002;137(2): 77–86.

15. Bliziotis IA, Michalopoulos A, Kasiakou SK, et al. Ciprofloxacin vs an aminoglycoside in combination with a beta-lactam for the treatment of febrile neutropenia: a meta-analysis of randomized controlled trials. Mayo Clin Proc 2005;80(9): 1146–56.

16. Pizzo PA, Hathorn JW, Hiemenz J, et al. A randomized trial comparing ceftazidime alone with combination antibiotic therapy in cancer patients with fever and neutropenia. N Engl J Med 1986;315(9):552–8.

17. Cometta A, Calandra T, Gaya H, et al. Monotherapy with meropenem versus combination therapy with ceftazidime plus amikacin as empiric therapy for fever in granulocytopenic patients with cancer. The International Antimicrobial Therapy Cooperative Group of the European Organization for Research and Treatment of Cancer and the Gruppo Italiano Malattie Ematologiche Maligne dell'Adulto Infection Program. Antimicrobial Agents Chemother 1996;40(5):1108–15.

18. Paul M, Borok S, Fraser A, et al. Additional anti-gram-positive antibiotic treatment for febrile neutropenic cancer patients. Cochrane Database Syst Rev 2005;3:CD003914.

19. Paul M, Borok S, Fraser A, et al. Empirical antibiotics against Gram-positive infections for febrile neutropenia: systematic review and meta-analysis of randomized controlled trials. J Antimicrob Chemother 2005;55:436–44.

20. Aoun M. Review: additional anti-gram-positive antibiotics do not reduce all-cause mortality in cancer and febrile neutropenia [comment]. ACP J Club 2006;144:3.

21. Freifeld A, Baden L, Brown A, et al. Fever and neutropenia. J Natl Compr Canc Netw 2004;2(5):390–432.

22. Clark O, Lyman G, Castro A, et al. Colony-stimulating factors for chemotherapy-induced febrile neutropenia: a meta-analysis of randomized controlled trials. J Clin Oncol 2005;23(18):4198–214.

23. Santolaya ME, Alvarez AM, Aviles CL, et al. Early hospital discharge followed by outpatient management versus continued hospitalization of children with cancer, fever, and neutropenia at low risk for invasive bacterial infection. J Clin Oncol 2004;22(18):3784–9.

24. Kamana M, Escalante C, Mullen CA, et al. Bacterial infections in low-risk, febrile neutropenic patients. Cancer 2005;104(2):422–6.
25. Stone P, Richardson A, Ream E, et al. Cancer-related fatigue: inevitable, unimportant and untreatable? Results of a multi-centre patient survey. Cancer Fatigue Forum. Ann Oncol 2000;11(8):971–5.
26. Mock V, Atkinson A, Barsevick A, et al. NCCN Practice Guidelines for Cancer-Related Fatigue. Oncology (Huntington) 2000;14:151–61.
27. Wang XS, Giralt SA, Mendoza TR, et al. Clinical factors associated with cancer-related fatigue in patients being treated for leukemia and non-Hodgkin's lymphoma. J Clin Oncol 2002;20(5):1319–28.
28. Groopman JE, Itri LM. Chemotherapy-induced anemia in adults: incidence and treatment. J Natl Cancer Inst 1999;91(19):1616–34.
29. Schrier S. Steensma D. Loprinzi C. Role of erythropoiesis-stimulating agents in the treatment of anemia in patients with cancer. Available at: www.uptodate.com. Accessed June 15, 2008.
30. Smith RE Jr, Aapro MS, Ludwig H, et al. Darbepoetin alpha for the treatment of anemia in patients with active cancer not receiving chemotherapy or radiotherapy: results of a phase III, multicenter, randomized, double-blind, placebo-controlled study. J Clin Oncol 2008;26(7):1040–50.
31. Perry M. Chemotherapy and liver disease. Available at: www.uptodate.com. Accessed June 15, 2008.
32. Benichou C. Criteria of drug-induced liver disorders. Report of an international consensus meeting. J Hepatol 1990;11(2):272–6.
33. Maria VA, Victorino RM. Development and validation of a clinical scale for the diagnosis of drug-induced hepatitis. Hepatology 1997;26(3):664–9.
34. Kawatani T, Suou T, Tajima F, et al. Incidence of hepatitis virus infection and severe liver dysfunction in patients receiving chemotherapy for hematologic malignancies. Eur J Haematol 2001;67(1):45–50.
35. Zuckerman E, Zuckerman T, Douer D, et al. Liver dysfunction in patients infected with hepatitis C virus undergoing chemotherapy for hematologic malignancies. Cancer 1998;83(6):1224–30.
36. Floyd J, Morgan J, Perry M. Cardiotoxicity of anthracycline-like chemotherapy agents. Available at: www.uptodate.com. Accessed June 15, 2008.
37. Vogelzang NJ. Nephrotoxicity from chemotherapy: prevention and management. Oncology (Huntington) 1991;5:97–102.
38. Ries F, Klastersky J. Nephrotoxicity induced by cancer chemotherapy with special emphasis on cisplatin toxicity. Am J Kidney Dis 1986;8:368–79.
39. Bressler RB, Huston DP. Water intoxication following moderate dose intravenous cyclophosphamide. Arch Intern Med 1985;145:548–9.
40. Merchan J. Chemotherapy and renal insufficiency. Available at: www.uptodate.com. Accessed June 15, 2008.
41. Cantrell JE Jr, Phillips TM, Schein PS. Carcinoma-associated hemolytic-uremic syndrome: a complication of mitomycin C chemotherapy. J Clin Oncol 1985;3: 723–34.
42. Yang H, Rosove MH, Figlin RA. Tumor lysis syndrome occurring after the administration of rituximab in lymphoproliferative disorders: high-grade non-Hodgkin's lymphoma and chronic lymphocytic leukemia. Am J Hematol 1999;62:247–50.
43. Sandler AB, Johnson DH, Herbst RS. Anti-vascular endothelial growth factor monoclonals in non-small cell lung cancer. Clin Cancer Res 2004;10: 4258S–62S.

44. Schrag D, Chung KY, Flombaum C, et al. Cetuximab therapy and symptomatic hypomagnesemia. J Natl Cancer Inst 2005;97:1221–4.
45. Belldegrun A, Webb DE, Austin HA 3rd, et al. Effects of interleukin-2 on renal function in patients receiving immunotherapy for advanced cancer. Ann Intern Med 1987;106:817–22.
46. Guleria AS, Yang JC, Topalian SL, et al. Renal dysfunction associated with the administration of high-dose interleukin-2 in 199 consecutive patients with metastatic melanoma or renal cell carcinoma. J Clin Oncol 1994;12:2714–22.
47. Ault BH, Stapleton FB, Gaber L, et al. Acute renal failure during therapy with recombinant human gamma interferon. N Engl J Med 1988;319(21):1397–400.
48. Anand AJ. Fluorouracil cardiotoxicity. Ann Pharmacother 1994;28:374–8.
49. Tolba KA, Deliargyris EN. Cardiotoxicity of cancer therapy. Cancer Invest 1999; 17:408–22.
50. Telli ML, Hunt SA, Carlson RW, et al. Trastuzumab-related cardiotoxicity: calling into question the concept of reversibility. J Clin Oncol 2007;25:3525–33.
51. Chu TF, Rupnick MA, Kerkela R, et al. Cardiotoxicity associated with tyrosine kinase inhibitor sunitinib. Lancet 2007;370:2011–9.
52. Vogelzang NJ, Frenning DH, Kennedy BJ. Coronary artery disease after treatment with bleomycin and vinblastine. Cancer Treat Rep 1980;64:1159–60.
53. Gilbert MR. The neurotoxicity of cancer chemotherapy. Neurologist 1998;4: 43–53.
54. Keime-Guibert F, Napolitano M, Delattre JY. Neurological complications of radiotherapy and chemotherapy. J Neurol 1998;245:695–708.
55. Wen PY. Central nervous system complications of cancer therapy. In: Schiff D, Wen PY, editors. Cancer neurology in clinical practice. Totowa (NJ): Humana Press; 2002. p. 287–326.
56. Lee JJ, Swain SM. Peripheral neuropathy induced by microtubule-stabilizing agents. J Clin Oncol 2006;24:1633–42.
57. Verstappen CC, Koeppen S, Heimans JJ, et al. Dose-related vincristine-induced peripheral neuropathy with unexpected off-therapy worsening. Neurology 2005; 64:1076–7.
58. Van den Bent MJ, Hilkens PH, Sillevis Smitt PA, et al. Lhermitte's sign following chemotherapy with docetaxel. Neurology 1998;50:563–4.
59. Wen P. Plotkin S. Neurologic complications of cancer chemotherapy. Available at: www.uptodate.com. Accessed July 15, 2008.
60. Phillips PC. Methotrexate toxicity. In: Rottenberg DA, editor. Neurological complications of cancer treatment. Boston: Butterworth-Heinemann; 1991. p. 115.
61. Walker RW, Allen JC, Rosen G, et al. Transient cerebral dysfunction secondary to high-dose methotrexate. J Clin Oncol 1986;4:1845–50.
62. Jardine LF, Ingram LC, Bleyer WA. Intrathecal leucovorin after intrathecal methotrexate overdose. J Pediatr Hematol Oncol 1996;18:302–4.
63. Spiegel RJ, Cooper PR, Blum RH, et al. Treatment of massive intrathecal methotrexate overdose by ventriculolumbar perfusion. N Engl J Med 1984;311: 386–8.
64. Widemann BC, Balis FM, Shalabi A, et al. Treatment of accidental intrathecal methotrexate overdose with intrathecal carboxypeptidase G2. J Natl Cancer Inst 2004;96:1557–9.
65. Sonis ST. The pathobiology of mucositis. Nat Rev Cancer 2004;4:277–84.
66. Sonis ST, Elting LS, Keefe D, et al. Perspectives on cancer therapy-induced mucosal injury: pathogenesis, measurement, epidemiology, and consequences for patients. Cancer 2004;100:1995–2025.

67. Keefe DM, Schubert MM, Elting LS, et al. Updated clinical practice guidelines for the prevention and treatment of mucositis. Cancer 2007;109:820–31.
68. National Cancer Institute Common Toxicity Criteria, version 3.0; 2003.
69. Peterson DE, Schubert MM. Oral toxicity. In: Perry MC, editor. The chemotherapy source book. 3rd edition. Baltimore (MD): Williams & Wilkins; 2001. p. 115–36.
70. Toljanic J. Bedard JF, Joyce R. Oral toxicity associated with chemotherapy. Available at: www.uptodate.com. Accessed July 15, 2008.
71. Dreizen S, Bodey GP, Valdivieso M. Chemotherapy-associated oral infections in adults with solid tumors. Oral Surg Oral Med Oral Pathol 1983;55:113–20.
72. Redding SW. Role of herpes simplex virus reactivation in chemotherapy-induced oral mucositis. NCI Monogr 1990;9:103–5.
73. Coda BA, O'Sullivan B, Donaldson G, et al. Comparative efficacy of patient-controlled administration of morphine, hydromorphone, or sufentanil for the treatment of oral mucositis pain following bone marrow transplantation. Pain 1997;72:333–46.
74. Alley E, Green R, Schuchter L. Cutaneous toxicities of cancer therapy. Curr Opin Oncol 2002;14:212–6.
75. Koon H. Drews R. Hypersensitivity reactions to systemic chemotherapy. Available at: www.uptodate.com. Accessed July 15, 2008.
76. Albanell J, Baselga J. Systemic therapy emergencies. Semin Oncol 2000;27:347–61.
77. Rahman A, Treat J, Roh JK, et al. A phase I clinical trial and pharmacokinetic evaluation of liposome-encapsulated doxorubicin. J Clin Oncol 1990;8:1093–100.
78. Leung WH, Lau JY, Chan TK, et al. Fulminant hyperpyrexia induced by bleomycin. Postgrad Med J 1989;65(764):417–9.
79. Payne A. Harris J. Savarese D. Chemotherapy extravasation injury. Available at: www.uptodate.com. Accessed July 15, 2008.
80. Fischer D, Knobf M, Durivage H. The cancer chemotherapy handbook. St Louis (MO): Mosby; 1997. p. 514.
81. Goolsby TV, Lombardo FA. Extravasation of chemotherapeutic agents: prevention and treatment. Semin Oncol 2006;33:139–43.
82. Dorr RT, Alberts DS. Vinca alkaloid skin toxicity: antidote and drug disposition studies in the mouse. J Natl Cancer Inst 1985;74:113–20.
83. Larson DL. Treatment of tissue extravasation by antitumor agents. Cancer 1982;49:1796–9.
84. Susser WS, Whitaker-Worth DL, Grant-Kels JM. Mucocutaneous reactions to chemotherapy. J Am Acad Dermatol 1999;40:367–98.
85. Wingard JR. Advances in the management of infectious complications after bone marrow transplantation. Bone Marrow Transplant 1990;6:371–83.
86. Wingard JR. Bacterial infections. In: Forman SJ, Blume KG, Thomas ED, editors. Hematopoietic cell transplantation. Boston: Blackwell Scientific; 1994. p. 537–49.
87. Wingard JR. Infections in allogeneic bone marrow transplant recipients. Semin Oncol 1993;20:80–7.
88. Anaissie E, Bodey GP, Kantarjian H, et al. Fluconazole therapy for chronic disseminated candidiasis in patients with leukemia and prior amphotericin B therapy. Am J Med 1991;91:142–50.
89. Abi-Said D, Anaissie E, Uzun O, et al. The epidemiology of hematogenous candidiasis caused by different Candida species. Clin Infect Dis 1997;24:1122–8.

90. Sable CA, Donowitz GR. Infections in bone marrow transplant recipients. Clin Infect Dis 1994;18:273–81.
91. Boyiadzis M, Gea-Benacloche J, Bishop M. Complications and follow-up after Hematopoietic Stem Cell Transplantation (HSCT). In: Boyiadzis M, Lebowitz P, Frame J, et al, editors. Hematology-oncology therapy. New York: McGraw-Hill; 2007. p. 674–93.
92. Harrington RD, Hooton TM, Hackman RC, et al. An outbreak of respiratory syncytial virus in a bone marrow transplant center. J Infect Dis 1992;165:987–93.
93. Ljungman P, Gleaves CA, Meyers JD. Respiratory virus infection in immunocompromised patients. Bone Marrow Transplant 1989;4:35–40.
94. Sparrelid E, Ljungman P, Ekelof-Andstrom E, et al. Ribavirin therapy in bone marrow transplant recipients with viral respiratory tract infections. Bone Marrow Transplant 1997;19:905–8.
95. Meyers JD. Fungal infections in bone marrow transplant patients. Semin Oncol 1990;17:10–3.
96. Enright H, Haake R, Weisdorf D, et al. Cytomegalovirus pneumonia after bone marrow transplantation. Risk factors and response to therapy. Transplantation 1993;55:1339–46.
97. Kadakia MP, Rybka WB, Stewart JA, et al. Human herpesvirus 6: Infection and disease following autologous and allogeneic bone marrow transplantation. Blood 1996;87:5341–54.
98. Yoshikawa T. Human herpesvirus 6 infection in hematopoietic stem cell transplant patients. Br J Haematol 2004;124:421–32.
99. Flomenberg P, Babbitt J, Drobyski WR, et al. Increasing incidence of adenovirus disease in bone marrow transplant recipients. J Infect Dis 1994;169:775–81.
100. Ochs L, Shu XO, Miller J, et al. Late infections after allogeneic bone marrow transplantation: comparison of incidence in related and unrelated donor transplant recipients. Blood 1995;86:3979–86.
101. Sullivan KM, Agura E, Anasetti C, et al. Chronic graft-versus-host disease and other late complications of bone marrow transplantation. Semin Hematol 1991;28:250–9.
102. Kawasaki H, Takayama J, Ohira M. Herpes zoster infection after bone marrow transplantation in children. J Pediatr 1996;128:353–6.
103. Couriel D, Caldera H, Champlin R, et al. Acute graft-versus-host disease: pathophysiology, clinical manifestations, and management. Cancer 2004;101:1936–46.
104. Schwartz JM, Wolford JL, Thornquist MD, et al. Severe gastrointestinal bleeding after hematopoietic cell transplantation, 1987-1997: incidence, causes, and outcome. Am J Gastroenterol 2001;96:385–93.
105. McDonald GB, Hinds MS, Fisher LD. Veno-occlusive disease of the liver and multiorgan failure after bone marrow transplantation: a cohort study of 355 patients. Ann Intern Med 1993;118:255–67.
106. Kumar S, DeLeve LD, Kamath PS, et al. Hepatic veno-occlusive disease (sinusoidal obstruction syndrome) after hematopoietic stem cell transplantation. Mayo Clin Proc 2003;78:589–98.

Caring for Patients with Malignancy in the Emergency Department: Patient–Provider Interactions

Tammie E. Quest, MD[a],*, Placid Bone, MD[b]

KEYWORDS

- Communication • Patient–doctor relationship • Caregiver
- Cancer • Spirituality • Breaking bad news

From 1997 to 2000, there were approximately 2.1 million cancer-related patient visits to US emergency departments (EDs).[1] The majority of the more than 1.2 million individuals with newly diagnosed cancer each year will experience significant distress during the course of their treatment. Of 28,777 patients over 65 years who died within 1 year of a diagnosis of lung, breast, or gastrointestinal cancer between 1993 and 1996, more than 9% had 1 or more ED visits in the last month of their life, and the number appears to be trending upward.[2] When patients with malignancy present to the ED, it is frequently as a result of physical distress but can be veiled with a patient or caregiver under stress. To optimize quality care, emergency clinicians should appreciate the unique complexities of a patient with cancer who is being cared for by the oncologists and be aware of the delicate dance that one must often perform to care for the patient in the ED, which not only allows a patient and the surrogates to express their needs but also enables clinicians to recognize where gaps and misunderstandings may be. This article focuses on discussing the patient–oncologist relationship, unique features of patients with advanced, metastatic cancer and their desire for treatment, paradoxes in advance care planning, and examination of patients and families under stress. Some tips for interacting with patients in whom an oncologic diagnosis is first established in the ED are also considered.

[a] Department of Emergency Medicine, Emory University School of Medicine, 69 Jesse Hill Jr. Drive, Atlanta, GA 30303, USA
[b] Interfaith Medical Center, 778 Lafayette Avenue, Brooklyn, NY 11221, USA
* Corresponding author.
E-mail address: tquest@emory.edu (T.E. Quest).

Emerg Med Clin N Am 27 (2009) 333–339
doi:10.1016/j.emc.2009.01.004
0733-8627/09/$ – see front matter. Published by Elsevier Inc.

emed.theclinics.com

ADVANCED CANCER AND CHEMOTHERAPY: THE NORM

The goal of chemotherapy in the context of metastatic disease is to prolong disease-free or overall survival, relieve symptoms, and improve quality of life. Chemotherapy has advanced significantly over the last decades, with decreasing toxicity and more lines of therapy for advanced stage disease. First-, second-, and even third-line chemotherapies have shown low toxicity and benefit in terms of survival and enhanced quality of life.[3,4] Oncologists struggle with the benefits of chemotherapy versus the burdens, particularly when the patient may be willing to accept risks for even a small potential benefit. Even when communication is clear and oncologists tell individuals that chemotherapy is not curative, patients and families report that they still believe that the chemotherapy has the ability to cure.[5] These patients, despite the oncologist's declaration that they have an incurable disease and are at the end of life, may still request aggressive cancer-directed therapy and refuse hospice and palliative care services.[6] Studies have shown that patients with cancer may be willing to accept cancer-directed therapies with significant morbidity and mortality and even experimental therapies with relatively high mortality for a "chance."[7]

THE PATIENT–ONCOLOGIST RELATIONSHIP

The emergency clinician most often closely works with the patient's oncologist, who directs the next steps in care. Similar to nephrologists, when a patient has advanced, metastatic disease, oncologists are often the direct care managers of the patient's complex problems, and the emergency clinician should be aware of this alliance. Oncologists are typically the managing physicians, and the patient, family, and caregivers often feel bonded to these clinicians even to the extent that the patient may feel that his or her life is in the clinician's hands. The oncologist determines the course of treatment and has the power to start and stop chemotherapy. For many patients living with serious, active cancer, chemotherapy may be viewed as the difference between life and death. Determinants of trust between the patient and oncologist include minimization of shame and humiliation, management of the power imbalance between doctor and patient without abuse or misuse; appreciation of how the patient is suffering from the experience of cancer, and an understanding of how the patient is suffering from the treatment provided by the oncologist.[8] Hope is the expectation of a positive outcome despite the circumstances.[9,10] Patients with incurable cancer can maintain hope in the face of incurable illness and want honesty, realism, as well as an individualized approach to communication from their oncologist.[11]

PARADOXES IN ADVANCE CARE PLANNING PREFERENCES IN PATIENTS WITH CANCER

Lamont and Siegler[12] demonstrated in their study of patients with cancer being admitted to the hospital that they (1) have advance care planning preferences and have discussed those preferences with family, and for unclear reasons, they neither share nor want their oncologist to know about their preferences; (2) over 50% of patients without an advance care plan at hospitalization would consider discussing them on the day of admission with hospital staff; and (3) patients closest to death were the least likely to report having an advance care plan. The observation of not sharing the advance care plan with the oncologist appears to be a unique finding in patients with cancer and is not found in patients with noncancer diagnosis. It has been postulated that discussing the advance care plan with the oncologist may interfere with "optimism" regarding treatment.[13]

PATIENTS AND FAMILIES UNDER STRESS

Factors that influence family coping include the following: past and current medical situation; family structure and roles; stage in the patient's life cycle; spirituality/faith; values and beliefs; patterns of communication and relating; socioeconomic factors/ resources; past experience with illness, disability, and death; and coping history and strengths.[14] It is impossible in one ED visit to assess all of the listed factors; however, the treating team may see one area or the other present itself as a dominant factor. There may be conflict in the family, particularly when the patient is declining rapidly, or there is additional stress on caregivers. Families that have suffered multiple losses or come from traditionally disadvantaged groups may also feel more vulnerable. The ED provider should be aware of the complexity of families, their coping mechanism, as well as the impact of internal and external influences.

INTERACTING WITH PATIENTS WITH CANCER IN THE EMERGENCY DEPARTMENT

The following points should be considered when interacting with patients, families, and caregivers of patients with oncologic disease in the ED (**Box 1**).

Reassure Patients and Caregivers that Physical Distress Will Be Relieved

Emergency clinicians should be explicit in their intent to relieve physical distress. Many patients and families fear that patients with cancer will suffer in pain or from other non-pain symptoms such as dyspnea, nausea, or vomiting. Lack of prompt attention to symptoms can cause extreme anxiety in patients and caregivers and rapidly dismantle trust between the patient and the ED team. Emergency clinicians should actively manage symptoms while searching for the underlying cause of the distress.

Use the ED Visit to Explore Coping

Patients and families may be scared of what may happen next and what might be expected. Inquiry into how the patient and family are currently coping can provide helpful insight into how to approach a patient and the caregivers. Living with cancer can be enormously stressful, and patients may be suffering from loss of function, loss of their role in the family, loss of relationships, and financial stress, and facing the end of life. A visit to the ED is a signal that there is physical or psychosocial distress that cannot be handled by the patient or caregiver. This may be something as medically straightforward as a fever while receiving chemotherapy but can be psychologically stressful to the patient or caregiver, as they worry about the ability to recover, progression of disease, fatigue related to hospitalization, or caregiver distress. Gauge how the patient and caregivers seem to react to information about the diagnosis and

---

Box 1
Interacting with a patient with cancer in the emergency department

- Reassure that pain and nonpain symptoms will be attended to
- Explore coping
- Explore goals of care/advance care planning
- Support the patient–oncologist relationship whenever possible
- Diffuse conflicts by finding common ground
- Be prepared to break bad news

treatment. Do they want full information? Is there some disconnect between the medical reality and their expectations? If so, what seems to be contributing to this? Establish whether the illness has had an impact on the patient's decision-making capacity, and, if not, consider whether or when it is likely to do so. Determine whether a proxy decision maker has been chosen. The emergency clinician can use the ED visit as an opportunity to initiate support services, such as pastoral care and social work or explore the need for spiritual or religious practices, which can be an important source of comfort and strength in dealing with illness and suffering. Any member of the ED team may initiate a simple spiritual assessment through a short spiritual screen such as the *FICA*[15] model, which uses 4 questions that examine *faith*, *influence*, *community*, as well as permission to further *address* these concerns (**Box 2**). A practitioner might use responses to this assessment to initiate spiritual care in the ED where available.

Explore the Patient's Goals of Care and Advance Care Planning Preferences

The evidence suggests that oncologists often do not discuss end of life with their patients,[16,17] and, ironically, cancer patients would prefer to discuss advance directives with someone other than their oncologists. Although emergency clinicians may feel somewhat sheepish in their approach to advance care planning with a cancer patient who states he or she has no advance care plan, they may in fact be initiating a much-wanted conversation. This can best be done by asking an open-ended question that deals with the hypothetical in the context of thresholds. For example, the emergency clinician might say *"Mr. Sims, it appears that this will not be an issue today, but in case you got much worse and you could no longer breathe on your own, have you ever thought about an artificial machine to sustain your life, such as a ventilator?"* If the patient answers, you might say, *"I encourage you to share that not only with your family and the doctors at the hospital but with your oncologist too."* These types of discussions may not solve the ED question of what the patient's end-of-life wishes are, but they may serve as a catalyst for planning, which may be facilitated with more information on a subsequent presentation.

Support the Patient's Oncologist and Encourage Communication between Both Parties

Although it can be difficult to be supportive of the patient and the oncologist when the emergency clinician feels that the oncologist may be overly optimistic, the emergency clinician can make an attempt to be supportive of the relationship between the patient and the oncologist. Some patients may insist that they do not want to know what is happening with their cancer.[18] Some cancer centers are helping to improve communication by providing physicians with scripts to discuss diseases with their patients as well as a checklist of questions for patients to ask of their clinicians. The emergency

---

Box 2
Assessing spirituality: the FICA model

Faith: "What things do you believe in that give meaning/purpose to your life?"

Importance/Influence: "What role do your spiritual beliefs play in regaining your health?"

Community: "Are you part of a religious or spiritual community?"

Address: "How would you like me to address these (spiritual) issues during your care and in this setting?"

physician may want to assist the patient's level of understanding regarding the disease and therapy with open-ended questioning, such as: *Tell me what your doctor has told you about what your treatments are doing. What did the doctor say regarding the ability of the treatment to manage the symptoms you have today, such as pain? Would you like me to ask your oncologist something when I can get him or her to discuss your case? Can I share with your oncologist what you have told me today?*

Diffuse the Difficult Interaction/Conflict by Finding Common Ground

Conflicts are common between patients and providers over such issues as treatment plan and disposition. Conflicts are often amplified when family members and the clinical care providers have different expectations. Differences can be amplified, and trust can be undermined when families and health care professionals come from backgrounds with different approaches. Although these differences are often personal, they may also take on greater meaning if they are perceived to be related to differences, thus creating a highly stressful atmosphere for everyone. Frustration can fuel anxiety and anger between health care professionals and family members during periods of conflict. Back and Arnold[19] have noted several pitfalls and the consequences of those pitfalls when dealing with conflict in palliative care settings. These are also applicable to the emergency setting and include the following:

- Avoiding or denying that a conflict exists
- Assuming that you know the whole story
- Repeatedly trying to convince the other party
- Assuming you know the other party's intentions
- Holding the other party responsible for fixing the issue
- Proceeding under the assumption that the issue can be resolved rationally or based on the evidence
- Declaring that the other party is ethically questionable
- Using anger or sarcasm as a coercive threat
- Ignoring one's own strong emotions
- Proceeding in the heat of the moment

Be Prepared to Break Bad News

Effective communication is an essential skill set for the emergency provider. The clinician must discuss diagnostic workup, treatment options, informed consent, and breaking bad news (eg, cancer recurrence, spread of disease) with patients and caregivers whom they have just met. Emergency providers are challenged with the task of communicating bad news in an understandable and empathetic manner. In the ED, time is limited and communication is compressed. The continuum of care takes place over hours not months or years as it does in the oncologist's office. The ED team approach is particularly helpful when communicating difficult news. The delivery of bad news is often seen as the physician's responsibility. Delivery of the actual news is only 1 part of the communication, however, and it should be remembered that the support that proceeds and follows this communication is critical. The entire ED team must work together to support patients, families, and one another during these disclosures. Several protocols exist for breaking bad news, and they all contain the same critical elements. Regardless of the protocol used, information should be delivered to the patient and families that are sensitive to their specific religious, cultural, and language needs. Physicians have a responsibility to make recommendations and guide families in accord with the family's decision-making preferences.[20] The SPIKES approach has been adapted from the work of Robert Buckman and others.

> **Box 3**
> **Breaking bad news (SPIKES Protocol)**
>
> *(S)etting*—Ensure privacy and confirm the facts of the case. Involve significant others, and sit down. Make a connection with the patient, and attempt to manage time constraints and interruptions in advance if possible
>
> *(P)atient's perception*—Ask for an initial impression of what the patient knows about his or her medical situation
>
> *(I)nvite patient to share*—Identify to whom the information should be given, and then ensure that the appropriate parties understand the findings
>
> *(K)nowledge translation*—Use plain and direct language to relay the information, and take time to formulate a prognosis. Do not minimize severity
>
> *(E)xplore emotions and show empathy*—Allow ample reaction time, and assure patients and caregivers that their reaction is normal. Remember the value of nonverbal communication
>
> *(S)ummarize and strategize*—Help the family process the new information and formulate next step plan

It was initially developed in an office-based setting and is concise enough to be an effective tool for communication in the emergency setting (**Box 3**).[21] Four common themes have emerged from research on giving bad news: sympathy of the news giver, clarity of the message, attitude of the news giver, and ability of the news giver to answer questions.[22] The seniority of the news giver was found to be relatively unimportant to most families, suggesting that the task should fall to the person able to spend the time to meet the family needs, provided this individual has adequate knowledge regarding the patient's clinical care and condition.

SUMMARY

Patients with cancer present to the ED with physical and psychosocial distress. The emergency clinician must be cognizant of the fact that patients with cancer are living longer and getting more aggressive therapies when the cancer is incurable, directed at optimization of symptoms and survival. Patients with cancer often have a difficult relationship with their oncologist, where hope and optimism hang in the balance, while the patient may show signs of decline. Ironically, patients may not want to discuss advance care planning with their oncologist, suggesting that emergency clinicians and other hospital-based clinicians may in fact be left with this task in crisis.

Above all, the emergency clinician should be able to reassure patients that pain and nonpain symptoms will be attended to promptly. The entire ED team (eg, registered nurse, nursing aid, chaplains, social workers) can explore goals of care, coping, and approach to advanced care planning. Respect should be given to the oncologist–patient relationship and this therapeutic relationship should be supported whenever possible. The emergency clinician should be willing to share with the oncologist areas to explore further with the patient or caregivers that have been identified in the ED as stress points. Finally, the emergency clinician should be prepared to break bad news in an empathic and supportive manner.

REFERENCES

1. Jemal A, Murray T, Samuels A, et al. Cancer statistics, 2003. CA Cancer J Clin 2003;53(1):5–26.

2. Earle CC, Neville BA, Landrum MB, et al. Trends in the aggressiveness of cancer care near the end of life. J Clin Oncol 2004;22(2):315–21.
3. Dancey J, Shepherd FA, Gralla RJ, et al. Quality of life assessment of second-line docetaxel versus best supportive care in patients with non-small-cell lung cancer previously treated with platinum-based chemotherapy: results of a prospective, randomized phase III trial. Lung Cancer 2004;43(2):183–94.
4. Shepherd FA, Rodrigues Pereira J, Ciuleanu T, et al. Erlotinib in previously treated non-small-cell lung cancer. N Engl J Med 2005;353(2):123–32.
5. Chow E, Andersson L, Wong R, et al. Patients with advanced cancer: a survey of the understanding of their illness and expectations from palliative radiotherapy for symptomatic metastases. Clin Oncol (R Coll Radiol) 2001;13(3):204–8.
6. Harrington SE, Smith TJ. The role of chemotherapy at the end of life: "when is enough, enough?" JAMA 2008;299(22):2667–78.
7. Matsuyama R, Reddy S, Smith TJ. Why do patients choose chemotherapy near the end of life? a review of the perspective of those facing death from cancer. J Clin Oncol 2006;24(21):3490–6.
8. Seetharamu N, Iqbal U, Weiner JS. Determinants of trust in the patient-oncologist relationship. Palliat Support Care 2007;5(4):405–9.
9. Hope. Available at: http://en.wikipedia.org/wiki/hope. Accessed July 26, 2008.
10. Silvestri G, Pritchard R, Welch HG. Preferences for chemotherapy in patients with advanced non-small cell lung cancer: descriptive study based on scripted interviews. BMJ 1998;317(7161):771–5.
11. Hagerty RG, Butow PN, Ellis PM, et al. Communicating with realism and hope: Incurable cancer patients' views on the disclosure of prognosis. J Clin Oncol 2005;23:1278–88.
12. Lamont EB, Siegler M. Paradoxes in cancer patients' advance care planning. J Palliat Med 2000;3(1):27–35.
13. Christakis NA. Death foretold: prophecy of prognosis and medical care. Chicago: University of Chicago Press; 1999.
14. Emanuel LL. Education in palliative and end of life care – trainer's guide. Psychosocial Module. 2005.
15. Puchalski CM, Romer AL. Taking a spiritual history allows clinicians to understand patients more fully. J Palliat Med 2000;3:129–37.
16. Koedoot CG, Oort FJ, de Haan RJ, et al. The content and amount of information given by medical oncologists when telling patients with advanced cancer what their treatment options are: palliative chemotherapy and watchful-waiting. Eur J Cancer 2004;40(2):225–35.
17. Sullivan AM, Lakoma MD, Matsuyama RK, et al. Diagnosing and discussing imminent death in the hospital: a secondary analysis of physician interviews. J Palliat Med 2007;10(4):882–93.
18. Neff P, Lyckholm L, Smith T. Truth or consequences: what to do when the patient doesn't want to know. J Clin Oncol 2002;20(13):3035–7.
19. Back AL, Arnold R. Dealing with conflict in caring for the seriously ill: "it was just out of the question." JAMA 2005;293(11):1374–81.
20. Rabow MW, Hauser JM, Adams J. Supporting family caregivers at the end of life. "They don't know what they don't know." JAMA 2004;4(291):483–91.
21. Buckman R. How to break bad news: a guide for health care professions. Baltimore (MD): Johns Hopkins University Press; 1992.
22. Jurkovich GJ, Pierce B, Pananed L, et al. Giving bad news: the family perspective. J Trauma 2000;5(48):865–70.

Treating Cancer Patients who Are Near the End of Life in the Emergency Department

Dawn Felch Rondeau, MS, ACNP, FNP[a,b,]*, Terri A. Schmidt, MD, MS[a]

KEYWORDS

- End of life • Cancer • Palliative care • POLST
- DNR • Decision-making capacity

Lydia is a 42-year-old woman with a diagnosis of metastatic leiomyosarcoma who comes to the emergency department with 1 week of increased fatigue. This fatigue is now so pronounced that she states, "I can no longer take care of myself." She is currently receiving palliative chemotherapy. Her hematocrit on presentation is 18. She is markedly pale, thin, tachypneic, and short of breath with any movement. She has a POLST form and does not wish to have resuscitation attempted, but she does want other limited interventions. How should the emergency care team proceed?

Patients with cancer seek care in the emergency department (ED) every day with a variety of symptoms and clinical presentations. These range from life-threatening events, such as impending respiratory failure, to fever, falls, medication side effects, or the always troublesome constipation.

Although cancer deaths, in general, have declined over the past years, ED visits for cancer-related emergencies are increasing. The 2005 National Hospital Ambulatory Medical Care Survey noted a decrease in cancer diagnoses from 0.8% in 1995 to 0.5% in 2005 but a 20% increase in ED visits.[1] The aging of America may be one of the reasons for the increase in both overall ED visits and visits related to cancer. The visit rates for patients aged 50 to 64 years increased 13%, and those aged 65 to 74 years increased by 11%. The Centers for Disease Control and Prevention estimates that by 2030 the number of Americans aged 65 years and older will more than double and represent 20% of the population![2] Daniel Murphy in "The Tsunami: Neither Hasten nor Postpone Death"[3] equates this increase in the baby boomer population as an incoming tsunami for the ED. This tsunami is set to overtake us with a tidal

[a] Department of Emergency Medicine, Oregon Health and Science University, 3181 S.W. Sam Jackson Park Road, Portland, OR 97239, USA
[b] Department of Nursing, Washington State University, Vancouver, WA 98686, USA
* Corresponding author. Department of Emergency Medicine, Oregon Health & Science University, 3181 S.W. Sam Jackson Park Road, Portland, OR 97239.
E-mail address: rondeaud@ohsu.edu (D.F. Rondeau).

Emerg Med Clin N Am 27 (2009) 341–354
doi:10.1016/j.emc.2009.01.006
0733-8627/09/$ – see front matter © 2009 Elsevier Inc. All rights reserved.

emed.theclinics.com

wave of patients, many of whom will have subspecialists involved with their care but no single individual practitioner responsible or knowledgeable about the entire person who can help in making decisions about end-of-life care. Patients with cancer, too, may arrive in the ED without a primary care provider who has been actively involved in their end-of-life planning. Unfortunately, at times, the goals of care will have to be determined at the time of the ED visit.

Efforts are underway to improve the care of patients near the end of life and honor their wishes in the emergency setting. In this article, we discuss some of the end-of-life issues related to patients with cancer coming to the ED, including those of legal documents, transmission of patient wishes, limiting factors in implementing those wishes, and the new horizon of palliative care in the ED.

THE NEED FOR IMPROVED END-OF-LIFE CARE PLANNING

In 1995, the results of the study to understand prognoses and preferences for outcomes and risks of treatments (SUPPORT) trial were published. This observational study followed by a controlled clinical trial was designed to improve end-of-life decision making and reduce the frequency of a prolonged process of dying.[4] It documented many shortcomings of end-of-life care. Although patients were seriously ill and their dying proved to be predictable, frequently discussions and decisions about do-not-resuscitate (DNR) status were not written until the last 2 days of life. In the controlled trial, an intervention was performed in which physicians were provided with reliable prognostic information as well as a nurse who initiated contact with the family, arranged meetings, provided forms so that the patient and family could participate in collaborative end-of- life decision making with the physician. The intent of the intervention was to initiate DNR discussions earlier, reduce pain and discomfort, as well as assist with resource use. This study revealed that despite the time of intensive intervention, there was no statistical change in these parameters.

Since the SUPPORT trial was reported, there has been increased discussion about end-of-life issues, with notable attempts to intervene, which vary from state to state and community to community. Although this article focuses on patients with cancer, the issues are not specific to a particular comorbidity or diagnosis. In the ED, we can anticipate that terminally ill patients will suddenly present at an end-of-life decision moment without preplanning.

Many, but not all, patients with cancer are in the later decades of life. Hamel and colleagues[5] reviewed previously published findings about how patients' age influenced their pattern of care. This study found that although older patients preferred less aggressive care than younger patients, many did want cardiopulmonary resuscitation (CPR). In contrast, their families and medical providers underestimated their desire for aggressive care. This was evidenced by lower hospital costs, decreased resource intensity, and higher rates of decisions to withhold life-sustaining treatments.[5] This study raises many societal and ethical issues with regard to the treatment of elders. There is no evidence that this large difference in cost was based on informed decisions by elders to decline treatment. In this study, patients aged 80 years and older had no difference in survival from that of their younger counterparts and were more likely to have a stable view of their desire for aggressive treatment.

ETHICAL BASIS FOR END-OF-LIFE CARE

Modern medicine has endorsed the ethical principles of beneficence, non-malfeasance, autonomy, and justice.[6] In most cases, Lo states the provider should follow 2 fundamental ethical guidelines: respecting patient autonomy and acting in the patient's best interest (beneficence).[7] A dilemma may occur when these 2 principles conflict. Beneficence presumes that providers will act in the patient's best interests and recommend treatments that are likely to provide benefit. When the patient's preferences are unknown and the patient cannot express preferences, the provider makes decisions based on what seems to be in the patient's best interest. Respect for patient autonomy assumes that a patient with decision-making capacity, who has been given information about a recommended plan of care, can consent to or refuse that plan and choose among other alternatives. This respect for autonomy also allows a patient with decision-making capacity to complete an advance directive that defines goals of care at a time when the patient can no longer speak for him or herself. These advance directives are often the basis for limiting or withholding life-sustaining interventions, but advance directives may also direct the health care system to "do everything." However, respect for autonomy has its limits. For example, respect for autonomy and beneficence conflict when patients (or their surrogates) want care or interventions that have no medical rationale in their situation or have already failed.

Respect for autonomy does not require offering futile treatments, although these have been hard to define, and the general public frequently has unrealistic expectations of survival. One study described a multimedia intervention to the general public to identify knowledge and personal preferences regarding resuscitation. Before the intervention, the public believed that 50% of patients would survive a cardiac arrest. In contrast, following the intervention, they recognized that only 16% would survive a cardiac resuscitation. The researchers note that further knowledge and teaching of the public are critical for their understanding and information-based decision making.[8]

Marco and colleagues[9] define as futile, interventions or therapies with a low expected likelihood of benefit to the patient and state that "physicians are under no ethical obligation to render treatments that they judge to have no realistic likelihood of medical benefit to the patient." However, these decisions should be made in the context of scientific evidence of likelihood of medical benefit, other benefits (including those that are intangible), potential risks of the proposed intervention, patient preferences, and family wishes. In many cases, however, there is reluctance to forgo treatment without clear practice standards, policy support for this decision, or concern about the legal ramifications.

In 2001, a panel was convened to look at end-of-life issues specific to cardiac care. The focus was on the ethics of cardiac care and guidelines for initiation of CPR. Additional topics reviewed were also advance directives and surrogate decision making, which are pertinent to our current topic.[10] Although acknowledging the ethical and cultural norms for ethical conduct, this panel focused on scientifically defined and proven data. These guidelines focused on data collection with regard to the likely positive outcome. In 1992, the cardiac guidelines included statements that CPR could be justifiably withheld or discontinued when no survivors had been reported under the same circumstances. In their review of this literature, no clinical criteria, *including metastatic cancer,* could predict a life-saving resuscitation or the futility of CPR.[11–13] A clinical decision rule to discern those who would survive an in-hospital cardiac arrest found that the survival was most dependent on whether the arrest was witnessed, what the initial cardiac rhythm was, the pulse response within the first 10 minutes, and whether the arrest was related to any comorbid conditions.[14]

DETERMINING THE GOALS OF CARE

When a patient with a life-threatening illness, such as cancer, first arrives in the ED, it is important to determine the patient's goals of care. Everyone involved in the patient's care, including the patient, the family, and the care team, will benefit from knowing these goals. For example, a patient with widely metastatic disease might be brought to the ED after a fall at home with a scalp laceration. A decision whether or not to obtain a head computed tomography scan might depend on whether or not the person would want any treatment for an acute intracranial process.

In determining the goals of care, it is often helpful to know and understand the trajectory of the patient's disease process. Dy and Lynn[15] identify three trajectories of illness to help anticipate or recognize what services may be needed:

- Progressive disability and eventual death over a period of weeks or a few months, often seen in patients with the most common solid malignancies: accounting for about 20% of the deaths after the age of 65 years.
- Slow decline with acute exacerbations and often a sudden death, most often due to chronic organ failure (eg, lung, kidney, or heart failure): about 25% of deaths after the age of 65 years.
- Long period of slow decline with worsening self-care ability: death often from an unpredictable intercurrent illness; the underlying condition is typically a chronic neurodegenerative disease, such as dementia: about 40% of deaths after the age of 65 years.

However, survival predictions are often inaccurate. A meta-analysis of terminally ill cancer patients showed that the median clinical prediction of survival was 42 days, when actual survival was 29 days.[16] It is, therefore, understandable how an established plan of care with a specific trajectory of interventions may fall short and require adjustment in the ED.

In some cases, patients will present to the ED unaware of their diagnosis or the anticipated trajectory of their illness. Most patients want to be informed whether their illness is now terminal. Others within the family group may not wish this fact disclosed.[13] Some fear that the patient will not continue to "fight" the illness or just give up if they are told of their now terminal diagnosis. These can be culturally based behaviors or a family-based culture that influences these perceptions.

In the best of situations, a patient and the family are in agreement with the treatment plan based on the diagnosis. Patients have identified that their preference is to die at home, surrounded by their family.[17] This family caregiving role, providing sometimes complex medical and nursing care to a family member, is not without considerable burden.[9,18,19] Clarifying treatment decisions can assist in early decision making, preventing unwanted interventions and relieve the burden of surrogates having to make difficult decisions without guidance.[20–22]

FUTILE TREATMENT INTERVENTIONS

As part of the discussion of goals of care, patients and families might seek treatments that are not reasonable under the circumstances. If there appears to be significant discordance in a plan regarding medically futile interventions, the Council on Ethical and Judicial Affairs of the American Medical Association has prepared a report[23] describing a process to resolve these issues using a consensus approach and additional resources within the hospital to work with the involved parties.

Although certain medical interventions may be considered to be futile, care should be taken in using the term with patients and families.[24] For example, short-term ventilator support, although futile in resolving the underlying disease process, may allow a patient to wake up and communicate with the family or allow a patient to survive to reach an important milestone, such as the graduation of a child. Alternatively, the family may wish to prolong life with any modality. The use of the word "futility" is commonly included in these discussions. If the goal is to return to the level of function before this illness, then futility would be an appropriate word. If however, the goal is not return to function but life extension, then it would not be futile.[23]

The initial conversation should involve the patient, proxy, and physician and begin the discussion about what constitutes futile care. The acceptable limits of intervention should be identified by the family group, within limits that are acceptable for the institution. If at this stage, it is clear that there is marked disagreement, the American Medical Association (AMA) report recommends an orderly transfer of care. Of course, this may be unrealistic in the ED and often the only option is to provide life-sustaining treatment until consensus can be reached.

The second step in the AMA process is joint decision making using any available outcome data and including the goals of treatment as identified by the patient and proxy. Ideally, this step is completed before the progression to a critical illness and the patient arrival in the ED.

The third step involves obtaining additional assistance, such as a consultant or patient representative, to help with resolution and facilitate the discussion. The role of this consultant is not to resolve the conflict or help make decisions but rather to facilitate the discussions to formulate consensus.

Finally, if the above steps are not successful in arbitrating a plan, an institutional committee such as an ethics committee, may be involved. This committee of course, must also include a manner for the proxy and patient to continue to have an equal and active role in this process.

The council further identified a fifth step if the institutional process agrees with the patient's desire but the physician remains unconvinced. The suggestion at that juncture is that the patient be transferred to another institution. In addition, if this group would agree with the provider's position but not with the patient and family, again the suggestion is for a transfer to another facility.

DECISION-MAKING ABILITY

Within the context of autonomy for patients is the assumption that the patient is able to make decisions. The capacity for making decisions includes the ability to receive, understand, and process information. It further requires the ability to make choices and communicate those choices. Larkin and Abbott further describe the need for intellect, memory, judgment, insight, language, attention, emotion, calculation, and expressive and receptive communication skills.[25,26]

In the ED, it is not uncommon to have difficulty assessing patients' decision-making ability in the context of stress, mental functioning at baseline, or pain. In the setting of acute disease, when immediate decisions need to be made, the American College of Emergency Physicians (ACEP) code of conduct states that "patients with decision making capacity must give their voluntary consent to treatment…and providers should be able to determine if a patient has decision-making capacity and who can act as a decision maker if the patient is unable to do so."[25] This may be harder than it seems.

There are a variety of standardized tests that may assist in this determination. These tests include questions assessing affect, calculation, attention, understanding, judgment, visual spatial, expressive, and receptive language skills, and memory. The Mini Mental State Examination has been extensively used and tested. However, standardized tests are time consuming and may not be readily available. The time-tested strategy of asking the patients to explain to the provider their understanding of the decision to be made and their personal decision is also validating of their cognition and understanding.

When impairment is evident, a surrogate decision maker will need to be identified. Surrogates are expected to make decisions on behalf of the individual on the basis of "substituted judgment" or what the patient would have wanted.[27] However, there is evidence that surrogates frequently do not know patient preferences. In one trial,[28] outpatients and their self-designated surrogate decision makers were randomized to 5 clinical scenarios. In one arm, the surrogates were asked to predict what the patients would have wanted without an advance directive, and in the other scenarios, this document was available to them. None of the scenarios with the benefit of an advanced directive helped the surrogate to make the same decision that the patient would have. However, it did improve the surrogates' perceived understanding and comfort.[28] A 2006 literature review reported 16 studies evaluating the accuracy of surrogate decision makers. In this review, one-third of the surrogates incorrectly predicted patients' end-of-life treatment preferences. Overall accuracy prediction was 68%.[29]

Coppola and colleagues compared the accuracy of surrogates as well as primary care providers, hospital-based physicians, and primary care physicians in making substituted judgments for elderly patients with and without advance directives. In this study, the family was still more accurate than physicians, and interestingly primary care physicians' accuracy was not improved with or without an advance directive. The predictions of hospital-based physicians were improved for some scenarios using an advance directive.[30]

In another scenario, a small group of patients and their surrogates were presented with 5 different scenarios. There was a high rate of discrepancy for treatment decisions in this group.[31] The best predictor of accurate surrogate decision making occurred in situations where a discussion had transpired between the patient and surrogate, particularly related to life-support issues.[32] Would patients be more interested in discussing end-of-life decisions if they were experiencing a disease that was now very severe? In a group of chronic lung disease patients, this question was studied. To the researcher's surprise, the patients did not appear any more or any less interested in discussing these issues than those who were earlier in their disease.[33,34]

Is there a better time to have these discussions? In looking at this issue in chronic lung disease patients, the severity of their illness, as determined by steroids, predicted forced expiratory volume, functional status score, recent hospitalizations, or recent mechanical ventilation, did not appear to have any relationship to their readiness or interest in discussion of end-of-life issues and planning.[33]

As previously noted, the SUPPORT trial[4] documented that many patients die without attention to these issues. Many providers have felt they lacked education or training that would assist in these conversations.[21] The AMA's Education for Physicians on End-of-Life Care (EPEC) curriculum provides that assistance focusing on skill development in this area.[34] EPEC has trained thousands of providers to improve their skills in end-of-life care. In 2005, the National Cancer Institute has founded a program, EPEC-EM, focused on training emergency care providers to increase their knowledge, comfort and skills in providing end-of-life care.

ADVANCE DIRECTIVES, DNR ORDERS AND POLST ORDERS

As part of the process of care planning and defining the goals of care, patients and their providers may complete advance directives and other documents that convey patient preferences. Advance directives are documents completed by the patients at the time in which they have decision-making capacity defining their treatment preferences at a future time when they may no longer be able to express their preferences. All 50 states and the District of Columbia have passed legislation on advance directives.[35]The Federal Patient Self-Determination Act of 1990 requires all facilities who accept Medicare or Medicaid to offer all patients information about advance directives, but this has resulted in only an estimated 15% to 20% of adults with advance directives.[27,36] On the other hand, patients near the end of life may be more likely to complete these forms. Bereaved family members report that completion of an advance directive resulted in less concerns about communication and increased use of hospice.[32,36]

The ACEP "Do Not Attempt Resuscitation (DNAR) in the Out-Of-Hospital Setting" emphasizes the importance of the out-of-hospital setting and the need for standard advance directives.[37] This position paper delineates that those with comorbid illness, terminal cancer and other irreversible disease states seldom survive a resuscitation effort. It recommends that the advance directive should include a plan of what to do for expected deaths, the use of 911, and that comfort care measures and palliative care measures are best provided by primary care providers and not Emergency Medical Services (EMS) system. It further stipulates that resuscitative measures should certainly be taken if a patient's wishes are unknown and that there needs to be an ideal identification device to communicate those wishes. These devices should be inclusive of a process, a list of surrogate decision makers and when and how to use them, the criteria for decision-making ability, and legal immunity provisions for those who use DNAR in good faith.

The initial attempt at providing directions for providers when the patient has lost decision-making capability included an advance directive commonly called the living will. This document included instructions about specific medical interventions with the ability to select parts or pieces of desired or not desired interventions. The living will document is helpful in describing continued medical care in case of loss of decision making resulting from injury or illness, however, it requires specific circumstances of the future illness and must be described accurately.[38] The living will may be useful in determining a treatment plan in the intensive care unit but is rarely useful in the ED, because it often has restrictive language, such as the requirement that a terminal condition be determined by 2 physicians and that there is no hope of survival.

Another document that may be more useful in the ED is the durable power of attorney for health care, which names a specific surrogate to make health care decisions for the patient when he or she is unable to make decisions. This mechanism allows for input from the provider team to the surrogate to analyze the wishes of the patient in real time and with real data. It, too, may be limited if the surrogate is not immediately available when decisions need to be made. Needless to say, the availability of these documents is critical to their implementation in the ED.[39–42]

Other documents seen in the ED include DNAR orders or the more comprehensive Physician Orders for Life-Sustaining Treatment (POLST). Unlike advance directives, DNAR orders and POLST are completed by a health care provider and are designed to turn patient preferences into actionable medical orders that apply at the present time. DNAR orders in the ED setting can be very helpful in directing care when a patient arrives in extremis, but the DNAR order applies only to a pulseless and apneic patient. There is evidence that many providers do not understand this limitation. One study found that many primary care providers believe that it also applies to intubation and cardioversion in patients who are not in cardiopulmonary arrest.[43] Further, a study in long-term care settings found a resuscitation attempt rate of 21% in patients with a DNAR order.[44]

POLST has been developed to address a number of the limitations of advance directives and DNR orders. In Oregon, a group of providers, EMS representatives, and long-term care providers began the development of a statewide program called the POLST. The group composition, format, and goal of the process were intentionally created to have a seamless movement of patients from one setting to another with their health care wishes transferring with them. It is a brightly colored document intended to stand out as posted on a refrigerator or within a patient's chart (**Fig. 1**). This form is divided into different areas to address resuscitation as well as a range of medical interventions. Choices can be made individually in each of these areas. This form is considered a medical order and can be signed in Oregon by a Doctor of Medicine or Doctor of Osteopathic Medicine physician, nurse practitioner or physician's assistant.[45] A review of the document by the National Quality Forum noted that "Compared with other advanced directives programs, POLST more accurately conveys end-of-life preferences and yields higher adherence by medical professionals."[46]

Two studies have been completed in long-term care settings and report that having a POLST form prevents unwanted life-sustaining treatments and hospitalization, and orders regarding resuscitation were usually followed. Unfortunately, the associated medical intervention orders were followed less consistently.[47,48] A study of a random sample of EMS personnel was completed to evaluate their experiences regarding the use of the POLST form.[40] In half of the cases where a POLST form was present, the EMS personnel used its direction to change the treatment plan, avoiding interventions that the patient did not want. Research was conducted and reported in 2004 regarding the implementation of this form in long-term care centers. About 71% of facilities in Oregon reported using this program for at least half of their residents. In an on-site review, these forms were present with DNR orders on 88% of the charts. The oldest old (85 years and older) were more likely than the young old (65–74 years) to have a DNR order.[49] Since the inception of POLST, it has been implemented in many other states (see www.POLST.org for states that currently have a POLST Paradigm Program) with continued acceptance and progression across the nation.

ROLE OF CULTURE

End-of-life discussions and approaches must occur in the context of ethnic and cultural differences. In discussing end-of-life issues, it would certainly be convenient to pull a reference to tell you specifically how to talk with a particular culture. For example, Muslim patients believe in the sanctity of life, however if treatment becomes futile, it is no longer mandatory.[50] In those who practice Tibetan Buddhism, practitioners are encouraged to practice death prayers for years before and at the time of death, and those in attendance should not be visibly upset but should be calm and maintain a meditative state of mind.[51] In a small study in a program focused on end-of-life issues in a Jewish population, the investigators were surprised by the variability of approaches to these issues. The variability included differences across the different branches of Judaism (ie, Orthodox or conservative) as well as family events (eg, history of family member who was a Holocaust survivor), all of which influenced the families' approach to end-of-life treatment.[52] Thomas and colleagues[53] reviewed the available research regarding preferences for end-of-life care in developed countries. The themes identified in this survey were life support, communication, decision making, and advance directives. This literature review of available research studies can provide a basis for discussing end-of-life care with a culturally sensitive approach.[53]

The discussion of difficulties across cultures would not be complete without mention of language differences and the difficulty in communication using interpreters (even sign language) to believe that what you are saying is being accurately interpreted

HIPAA PERMITS DISCLOSURE TO HEALTH CARE PROFESSIONALS AS NECESSARY FOR TREATMENT

Physician Orders
for Life-Sustaining Treatment (POLST)

First follow these orders, then contact physician, NP, or PA. These medical orders are based on the person's current medical condition and preferences. Any section not completed does not invalidate the form and implies full treatment for that section.

Last Name/ First/ Middle Initial

Address

City / State / Zip

Date of Birth (mm/dd/yyyy) | Last 4 SSN | Gender ☐ M ☐ F

A
Check One

CARDIOPULMONARY RESUSCITATION (CPR): Person has no pulse __and__ is not breathing.

☐ Attempt Resuscitation/CPR   ☐ Do Not Attempt Resuscitation/DNR (Allow Natural Death)

When not in cardiopulmonary arrest, follow orders in **B**, **C** and **D**.

B
Check One

MEDICAL INTERVENTIONS: Person has pulse and/__or__ is breathing.

☐ **Comfort Measures Only** Use medication by any route, positioning, wound care and other measures to relieve pain and suffering. Use oxygen, suction and manual treatment of airway obstruction as needed for comfort. *Do not transfer to hospital for life-sustaining treatment. Transfer if comfort needs cannot be met in current location.*

☐ **Limited Additional Interventions** Includes care described above. Use medical treatment, IV fluids and cardiac monitor as indicated. Do not use intubation, advanced airway interventions, or mechanical ventilation. May consider less invasive airway support (e.g. CPAP, BiPAP). *Transfer to hospital if indicated. Avoid intensive care.*

☐ **Full Treatment** Includes care described above. Use intubation, advanced airway interventions, mechanical ventilation, and cardioversion as indicated. *Transfer to hospital if indicated. Includes intensive care.*

Additional Orders: _____

C
Check One

ANTIBIOTICS

☐ No antibiotics. Use other measures to relieve symptoms.
☐ Determine use or limitation of antibiotics when infection occurs.
☐ Use antibiotics if medically indicated.

Additional Orders: _____

D
Check One

ARTIFICIALLY ADMINISTERED NUTRITION: Always offer food by mouth if feasible.

☐ No artificial nutrition by tube.
☐ Defined trial period of artificial nutrition by tube.
☐ Long-term artificial nutrition by tube.

Additional Orders: _____

E

REASON FOR ORDERS AND SIGNATURES

My signature below indicates to the best of my knowledge that these orders are consistent with the person's current medical condition and preferences as indicated by the **discussion with**:

☐ Patient ☐ Health Care Representative ☐ Parent of Minor

☐ Court-Appointed Guardian ☐ Other _____

Print Primary Care Professional Name	Office Use Only
Print Signing Physician / NP / PA Name and Phone Number ( )	
Physician / NP / PA Signature (mandatory) Date	

SEND FORM WITH PERSON WHENEVER TRANSFERRED OR DISCHARGED

© CENTER FOR ETHICS IN HEALTH CARE, Oregon Health & Science University. 3181 Sam Jackson Park Rd, UHN-86, Portland, OR 97239-3098 (503) 494-3965

Fig. 1. Oregon Physician Orders for Life-Sustaining Treatment (POLST) form. (*Courtesy of* the Center for Ethics in Health Care, Oregon Health & Science University, Portland, OR; with permission.)

and in a manner that is culturally competent. Minority cultural groups often believe they are treated differently, and they do not trust providers who use unclear terms, with perceived negative attitudes toward them.[54]

Therefore, although it is certainly helpful to have the context of a culture or ethnic heritage, the truth is that each family and situation has its own values and communication patterns that may be inclusive of that heritage but are different and unique to the individual and the family. In end-of-life discussions, the challenge is to incorporate these subtle and important variables.

PALLIATIVE CARE IN THE ED

Patients who present to the ED with cancer are often seeking assistance with symptom control and not usually diagnosis or treatment of their underlying disease. Palliative care is designed to emphasize care and symptom control rather than cure.[55–57] The definition of palliative care includes medical care focused on relief of physical, emotional, and existential suffering and support for the best possible quality of life for patients and their family caregivers.[58] Palliative care developed from the roots of the hospice movement in the 1970s in the United States. It differs from hospice care in that hospice is available only to the terminally ill (death is likely within 6 months). Palliative care is available to patients with advanced chronic disease who are not eligible for hospice benefits. The World Health Organization (WHO) components of palliative care are summarized in **Box 1**.[59]

Solano and colleagues[60] in their review of cancer patients as well as those with chronic obstructive pulmonary disease (COPD), renal disease, acquired immunodeficiency syndrome, and heart failure, found a similar constellation of symptoms at end of life. Pain and fatigue were present in more than 50% of the patients, whereas breathlessness was most common in those with heart failure or COPD.

Pain, of course, is the most concerning symptom and was present in 35% to 95% of the cancer patients.[60] Additional symptoms specific to cancer included lack of energy (69%), weakness (60%), and appetite loss (53%). In the last 2 weeks of life, weight loss (86%) was more prevalent, whereas pain (45%), nausea (17%), and urinary symptoms (6%) were less frequent.[61]

The focus on methods of symptom relief and comfort care, including pain relief and treatment of symptoms, such as shortness of breath, nausea and vomiting, anxiety and constipation, is an important aspect of the treatment of patients with cancer in the ED. Recently, the American Board of Emergency Medicine joined with other specialty boards to create subspecialty board certification in palliative care, recognizing this area as requiring additional training and expertise. A systematic review delineating the evidence for effective interventions to improve end-of-life care has been completed by Lorenz and colleagues.[62] The recommendations include the prescription of pain medications, oxygen, antidepressant drugs, and psychological treatments. In 2008, The British Medical Journal Group published an evidence-based review covering symptom assessment and management.[63] Specific treatment strategies particularly focused on pain management are discussed elsewhere in this issue.

Caregivers of patients with cancer may also be in distress at the time they come to the ED. Aoun and colleagues[63] reviewed the literature regarding the extent of physical and psychosocial morbidity and economic disadvantage that home palliative care providers suffer as a result of their caregiver role. The influence of sleep loss and the role it plays in depression among caregivers have also been studied.[64,65]

Box 1
WHO components of palliative care

- To regard death as part of life and a normal process
- Neither hasten nor delay death
- To use a team approach to address the needs of patients and their families, including bereavement
- To initiate palliative care early in a patient's illness, even when he or she is still receiving life-prolonging treatments, such as chemotherapy or radiation therapy

The lack of control over their own lives and their personal routines along with a financial burden reported to be 10% of their total income is a major issue in the stressors associated with this role.[66,67] ED providers may be able to help by providing needed family support. One study found that the key ingredients to success as a caregiver were the patient's illness experience, the caregiver's relationship with this patient, and the patient's recognition of the caregiver's contribution to the care.[68]

Ideally, all patients with a serious illness should talk with their family, friends, and physician about their goals and values and how they would like those to be considered in light of their illness. As providers, we need to recognize that when these patients are being seen in the ED this may be an excellent time to review their plan of care. Is there a new symptom or disease progression that may change their plan? Is this the time to talk specifically about desired or undesired interventions?

SUMMARY

At times, there is a tendency to see the ED visit as a failure in planning for disease progression and anticipatory planning for symptom management or a failure of the caregivers to cope. Some might see the ED visit as a failure of the primary provider or team to anticipate the end-of-life needs of patients; however, disease progression and symptom management is not a static or numerically predictive science. We need to see such visits as an opportunity to further refine and modify the plan of care and to incorporate elements of palliative care into the plan. As Malin states in the title of her article, "Bridging the Divide: Integrating Cancer-Directed Therapy and Palliative Care," we should not be choosing one or the other but rather incorporating interventions and therapies from each.[69]

In the analogy of a vessel as life, Schmidt is articulate in the illumination of the patient as an entire vessel. This vessel may develop some cracks, particularly as death approaches. These cracks and their timing are not easily predictable. In the case of a vessel cracking, the easing of pain and suffering within the patients' realm of family, faith, community, and meaning should be our primary goal.

The ED will continue to be an available resource for palliative care treatment. The challenge is to create the knowledge base, communication systems, physical support, and staffing within the environment so that we can provide excellent care for end-of-life patients.

REFERENCES

1. Nawar EW, Niska RW, Xu J. National hospital ambulatory medical care survey: 2005 emergency department summary. In: VAH, editor. Statistics, vol. 386. U.S. Department of Health and Human Services. Centers for Disease Control and Prevention, National Center for Health Statistics; 2007. p. 1–32.
2. Centers for Disease Control and Prevention and the Merck Company Foundation. The State of Aging and Heatlh in America 2007. Available at: www.cdc/gov/aging. Accessed May 12, 2008.
3. Murphy DG. The Tsunami: neither hasten nor postpone death. Emergency Medicine News 2004;26(13):14–6.
4. The SUPPORT Principal Investigators. A controlled trial to improve care for seriously ill hospitalized patient: the study to understand prognoses and preferences for outcomes and risks of treatments (SUPPORT). JAMA 1995;274(20):1591–8.
5. Hamel MF, Lynn J, Teno JM, et al. Age-related differences in care preferences, treatment decisions, and clinical outcomes of seriously ill hospitalized adults: lessons from SUPPORT. J Am Geriatr Soc 2000;48(5):176–82.

6. Beachamp TL, CJ. Principles of biomedical ethics. 5th edition. New York: Oxford University Press; 2001.

7. Lo B. Ethical issues in clinical medicine. In: Braunwald EF, Anthony, Kasper Dennis, editors. Introduction to clinical medicine. 15th edition. Columbus (OH): McGraw-Hill; 2001. p. 5–8.

8. Marco CA, Larkin GL. Public education regarding resuscitation: effects of a multi-media intervention. Ann Emerg Med 2003;42(2):256–60.

9. Marco CA, Larkin GL, Moskop JC, et al. Determination of "futility" in emergency medicine. Ann Emerg Med 2000;35:604–12.

10. Abramson ND, de Vos R, Fallat ME, et al. Ethics in emergency cardiac care. Ann Emerg Med 2001;37(4):S196–200.

11. Bowker L, Stewart K. Predicting unsuccessful cardiopulmonary resuscitation (CPR): a comparison of three morbidity scores. Resuscitation 1999;40:89–95.

12. Ebell MH, Kruse JA, Smith M, et al. Failure of a three decision rule to predict the outcome of in-hospital cardiopulmonary resuscitation. Med Decis Making 1997; 17:171–7.

13. Vitelli CE, Cooper K, Rogatko A, et al. Cardiopulmonary resuscitation and the patient with cancer. J Clin Oncol 1991;9:111–5.

14. van Walraven C, Forster AJ, Parish DC, et al. Validation of a clinical decision aid to discontinue in-hospital cardiac arrest resuscitations. JAMA 2001;285(12): 1602–6.

15. Dy S, Lynn J. Getting services right for those sick enough to die. BMJ 2007;334: 511–3.

16. Glare P, Virik K, Jones M, et al. A systematic review of physicians' survival predictions in terminally ill cancer patients. BMJ 2003;327:195–8.

17. Higginson IJ, Sen-Gupta GJ. Place of care in advanced cancer: a qualitiative systematic literature review of patient preferences. J Palliat Med 2000;3(3): 287–300.

18. Haley WE, LaMonde LA, Han B, et al. Family caregiving in hospice: effects on psychological and health functioning among spousal caregivers of hospice patients with lung cancer or dementia. Hosp J 2001;15(4):1–18.

19. McCorkle R, Pasacreta JV. Enhancing caregiver outcomes in palliative care. Cancer Control 2001;8(1):36–45.

20. Fischer GS, Arnold RM, Tulsky JA. Talking to the older adult about advance directives. Clin Geriatr Med 2000;16:239–54.

21. Emanuel LL, Danis M, Pearlman RA, et al. Advance care planning as a process: structuring the discussions in practice. J Am Geriatr Soc 1995;43:440–6.

22. Huggins M, Brooks L. Discussing end-of-life care with older patients: what are you waiting for? Geriatr Aging 2007;10(7):461–4.

23. Affairs CoEaJ. Medical futility in end-of-life care: report of the council on Ethical and judicial affairs 1999.

24. Gillick MR, HP, Connor RF, editors. Ethical issues near the end of life. UpToDate; 2008. Available at: www.uptodate.com. Accessed May 12, 2008.

25. Larkin G. A code of conduct for academic emergency medicine. Acad Emerg Med 1999;6:45.

26. Larkin GL, Marco CA, Abbott JT. Emergency determination of decision-making capacity: balancing autonomy and beneficence in the emergency department. Acad Emerg Med 2001;8:282–4.

27. Gillick MR. Advance care planning. N Engl J Med 2004;350(1):7–8.

28. Ditto PH, Danks JH, Smucker WD, et al. Advance directives as acts of communication: a randomized controlled trial. Arch Intern Med 2001;161(3):421–30.

29. Shalowitz DI, Garrett-Mayer E, Wendler D. The accuracy of surrogate decision makers: a systematic review. Arch Intern Med 2006;166:493–7.
30. Coppola KM, Ditto PH, Danks JH, et al. Accuracy of primary care and hospital-based physicians' predictions of elderly outpatients' treatment preferences with and without advance directives. Arch Intern Med 2001;161(3):431–40.
31. Hare J, Pratt C, Nelson C. Agreement between patients and their self-selected surrogates on difficult medical decisions. Arch Intern Med 1992;152(5):1049–54.
32. Suhl J, Simons P, Reedy T, et al. Myth of substituted judgement. Surrogate decision making regarding life support is unreliable. Arch Intern Med 1994; 154(1):90–6.
33. Pfeifer MP, Mitchell CK, Chamberlain L. The value of disease severity in predicting patient readiness to address end-of-life issues. Arch Intern Med 2003;163: 609–12.
34. Emanuel LL, VGC, Ferris FD. Education for physicians on end-of-life care trainer's guide: EPEC project. The Robert Wood Johnson Foundation: Institute for Ethics at the American Medical Association; 1999.
35. Quest TE, AJ. Palliative care and the emergency physician: finding our way. SAEM Newsl 2003;15(4):14. Available at: www.acep.org. Accessed May 12, 2008.
36. Teno JM, Gruneir A, Schwartz Z, et al. Association between advance directives and quality of end-of-life care: a national study. J Am Geriatr Soc 2007;55: 189–94.
37. American College of Emergency Physicians. Do Not Attempt Resuscitation (DNAR) in the Out-Of-Hospital Setting Policy Paper. Available at: www.acep.org/practres; 2008;1–4. Accessed April 1, 2008.
38. Chang TT, Schecter WP. Injury in the elderly and end-of- life decisions. Surg Clin North Am 2007;87:229–45.
39. Iserson K. A simplitified prehospital advance directive law: Arizona's approach. Ann Emerg Med 1993;22(11):1703–10.
40. Schmidt TA, Hickman SE, Tolle SW, et al. The physician orders for life-sustaining treatment (POLST) program: Oregon emergency medical technicians' practical experiences and attitudes. J Am Geriatr Soc 2004;52:1430–4.
41. Morrison RS, Olson E, Mertz KR. The inaccessibility of advance directives on transfer from ambulatory to acute care settings. JAMA 1995;274:478–82.
42. Lahn M, Friedman B, Bijur P, et al. Advance directives in skilled nursing facility residents transferred to emergency departments. Acad Emerg Med 2001;8(12): 1158–62.
43. Lerner E, Billittier AJ, Hallinan K. Out-of-hospital do-not-resuscitate orders by primary care physicians. J Emerg Med 2002;23(4):425–8.
44. Becker LJ, Yeargin K, Rea TD, et al. Resuscitation of residents with do not resuscitate orders in long-term care facilities. Prehosp Emerg Care 2003;7(3):303–6.
45. Center for Ethics in Health Care OHSU. Available at: http://www.POLST.org. Accessed June 8, 2008.
46. Forum NQ. A Framework and preferred Practices for Palliative and Hospice Care Quality. A Consensus Report: Washington, DC; 2006.
47. Tolle SW, Tilden VP, Nelson CA, et al. A prospective study of the efficacy of the physician order form for life-sustaining treatment. J Am Geriatr Soc 1998;46(9): 1097–102.
48. Lee MA, Brummel-Smith K, Meyer J, et al. Physician orders for life-sustaining treatment (POLST): outcomes in a PACE program. Program of all-inclusive care for the elderly. J Am Geriatr Soc 2000;48(10):1219–25.

49. Hickman SE, Tolle SW, Brummel-Smith K, et al. Use of the Physician Orders for Life-Sustaining Treatment Program in Oregon Nursing Facilities: beyond resuscitation status. J Am Geriatr Soc 2004;52:1424–9.

50. Lawrence P, Rozmus C. Culturally sensitive care of the Muslim patient. J Transcult Nurs 2001;12(3):228–33.

51. Smith-Stone M. End-of-life needs of patients who practice Tibetan Buddhism. Am J Hosp Palliat Nurs 2005;7(4):228–33.

52. Bonura D, FM, Roesler M, et al. Culturally congruent end-of-life care for Jewish patients and their families. J Transcult Nurs 2001;12(3):211–20.

53. Thomas R, WD, Justic C, et al. A literature review of preferences for end-of-life care in developed countries in individuals with different cultural affiliations and ethnicity. Am J Hosp Palliat Nurs 2008;10(3):1–16.

54. Valente S, HB, Anderson, et al. Culturally Diverse Communities and End-of-Life Care. Accessed June 12, 2008.

55. Derse A. The emrgency physician and end-of-life care. Virtual Mentor 2001;3(4):1–3 Available at: http://virtualmentor.ama-assn.org/2001/04. Accessed April 1, 2008.

56. DeSandre PL. Handling emergencies in the palliative phase of care. Emerg Med 2007;30–6.

57. Nantawadee PL, Washington G. Management of common symptoms at end of life in acute-care settings. Int J Nurs Pract 2008;8(8):610–5.

58. Brunnhuber K, NS, Meier DE, et al. Putting evidence in to practice: palliative care vol. 1. BMJ Publishing Group 2008.

59. World Health Organization. Cancer control: knowledge into action: WHO guide for effective programmes: module 5: palliative care. Available at: http://www.who.int/cancer/media/FINAL-Palliative%20Care%20Module.pdf; 2007. Accessed April 1, 2009.

60. Solano JP, Gomes B, Higginson IJ. A comparison of symptom prevalence in far advanced cancer, AIDS, heart failure, chronic obstructive pulmonary disease, and renal disease. J Pain Symptom Manage 2006;31:58–69.

61. Teunissen SC, Wesker W, Kruitwagen C, et al. Symptom prevalence in patients with incurable cancer: a systematic review. J Pain Symptom Manage 2007;34:94–104.

62. Lorenz KA, Lynn J, Dy SM, et al. Evidence of improving palliative care at the end of life: a systematic review. Ann Intern Med 2008;148:147–59.

63. Aoun SM, Kristjanson LJ, Currow DC, et al. Caregiving for the terminally ill: at what cost? Palliat Med 2005;19:551–5.

64. Carter P. Family Caregivers' sleep loss and depression over time. Cancer Nurs 2003;26(4):253–9.

65. Farber SJ, Egnew TR, Herman-Bertsch JL, et al. Issues in end-of-life care: patient, caregiver and clinician perceptions. J Palliat Med 2003;6(1):19–31.

66. Emanuel EJ, Fairclough DL, Slutsman J, et al. Understanding economic and other burdens of terminal illness: the experience of patients and their caregivers. Ann Intern Med 2000;132:451–9.

67. Stajduhar KI, Martin WL, Barwich D, et al. Factors influencing family caregivers' ability to cope with providing end-of-life cancer care at home. Cancer Nurs 2008;31(1):77–85.

68. Malin J. Bridging the divide: integrating cancer-directed therapy and palliative care. J Clin Oncol 2004;22(17):3438–40.

69. Schmidt T. Futility futilis—the leaky vessel. Ann Emerg Med 2000;35:615–7.

Index

Note: Page numbers of article titles are in **boldface** type.

A

Emerg Med Clin N Am 27 (2009) 355–362
doi:10.1016/S0733-8627(09)00048-0
0733-8627/09/$ – see front matter © 2009 Elsevier Inc. All rights reserved.

emed.theclinics.com

Moving?

Make sure your subscription moves with you!

To notify us of your new address, find your **Clinics Account Number** (located on your mailing label above your name), and contact customer service at:

E-mail: elspcs@elsevier.com

800-654-2452 (subscribers in the U.S. & Canada)
314-453-7041 (subscribers outside of the U.S. & Canada)

Fax number: 314-523-5170

Elsevier Periodicals Customer Service
11830 Westline Industrial Drive
St. Louis, MO 63146

*To ensure uninterrupted delivery of your subscription, please notify us at least 4 weeks in advance of move.

Printed and bound by CPI Group (UK) Ltd, Croydon, CR0 4YY

08/06/2025

01896873-0013